Breeder's Club

Secrets to Multiple Loads

Amber Creame

ISBN: 9781778905421
Imprint: Telephasic Workshop
Copyright © 2024 Amber Creame.
All Rights Reserved.

Contents

Introduction 1
The Erotic Lifestyle Guide Explained 1

Understanding Breeding Scenes 15
Defining Breeding Scenes 15

Preparing for Breeding Scenes 27
Communication and Negotiation 27

Creating the Perfect Breeding Environment 41
Setting the Scene 41

Techniques for Maximizing Pleasure 55
Foreplay and Teasing 55

Bibliography 63

Mastering Multiple Loads 69
Understanding Male Anatomy 69

Strategies for Managing Multiple Participants 83
Solo Breeding 83

Safety and Consent in Breeding Scenes 99
Establishing and Maintaining Consent 99

Exploring Power Dynamics in Breeding Scenes 113
Dominance and Submission 113

Beyond the Bedroom: Breeding in Public and Group Settings 127

Public Breeding Scenes 127

Mental and Emotional Well-being in Breeding Scenes 141
Processing and Aftercare 141

Conclusion 153
Embracing the Breeding Lifestyle 153

Bibliography 169

Resources 171
Recommended Reading 171
Online Communities and Support Groups 183
Professional Services 196

Index 209

Introduction

The Erotic Lifestyle Guide Explained

What is an Erotic Lifestyle Guide?

An Erotic Lifestyle Guide serves as a comprehensive resource designed to educate, inspire, and empower individuals and couples to explore their sexual desires and fantasies in a safe and consensual manner. It encompasses a wide array of topics, from practical advice to theoretical frameworks, all aimed at enhancing the erotic experience.

At its core, an Erotic Lifestyle Guide is not merely a manual on sexual techniques; it is an invitation to delve deeper into the complexities of human sexuality. It encourages readers to embrace their desires while fostering an understanding of the emotional, psychological, and relational dynamics involved in erotic exploration.

Theoretical Frameworks

The foundation of an Erotic Lifestyle Guide is built upon several key theoretical frameworks that inform our understanding of human sexuality. These include:

1. **Kinsey's Continuum of Sexual Orientation**: This theory posits that sexual orientation exists on a spectrum rather than as a binary classification. This perspective encourages individuals to explore their desires without the constraints of societal labels.

2. **The Sexual Response Cycle**: Proposed by Masters and Johnson, this model outlines the stages of sexual arousal, plateau, orgasm, and resolution. Understanding this cycle can help individuals and couples navigate their experiences more effectively.

3. **Attachment Theory**: This psychological framework explores how different attachment styles influence relationships and intimacy. Recognizing one's

attachment style can enhance communication and emotional connection during erotic exploration.

4. **Consent and Communication Models**: The importance of clear, informed consent and effective communication cannot be overstated. Models such as the FRIES acronym (Freely given, Reversible, Informed, Enthusiastic, Specific) provide a framework for understanding and practicing consent in erotic contexts.

Common Problems Addressed

An Erotic Lifestyle Guide addresses several common problems that individuals and couples may encounter on their sexual journeys:

- **Miscommunication**: Many couples struggle with expressing their desires, leading to misunderstandings and dissatisfaction. This guide emphasizes the importance of open dialogue and negotiation to foster intimacy and connection.

- **Fear of Judgment**: Societal norms often instill fear of judgment regarding sexual preferences. The guide encourages readers to embrace their fantasies without shame, promoting a healthy exploration of sexuality.

- **Safety Concerns**: Engaging in erotic activities can raise concerns about physical and emotional safety. The guide provides practical advice on establishing boundaries, safe words, and aftercare practices to ensure a positive experience.

- **Lack of Knowledge**: Many individuals feel uninformed about various sexual practices, leading to missed opportunities for pleasure. This guide aims to educate readers on techniques, anatomy, and strategies to enhance their erotic experiences.

Examples of Content

An Erotic Lifestyle Guide encompasses a diverse range of content, including:

- **Practical Techniques**: Step-by-step instructions on various sexual practices, such as massage, oral techniques, and role-play scenarios, designed to enhance pleasure and intimacy.

- **Personal Narratives**: Anecdotes and testimonials from individuals who have explored their erotic desires, providing relatable insights and inspiration.

- **Workshops and Exercises**: Interactive activities that encourage couples to practice communication, negotiation, and exploration of fantasies in a structured manner.

- **Resources for Further Exploration**: Recommendations for books, articles, and online communities that support ongoing learning and connection with like-minded individuals.

Conclusion

In summary, an Erotic Lifestyle Guide is a multifaceted resource that empowers individuals and couples to explore their sexual desires in a safe and informed manner. By blending theoretical insights with practical advice, it offers a holistic approach to enhancing erotic experiences. Whether one is new to the world of erotic exploration or seeking to deepen their understanding, this guide serves as a valuable companion on the journey toward sexual fulfillment and connection.

Why Breeding Scenes?

Breeding scenes, often shrouded in layers of taboo and intrigue, represent a profound intersection of fantasy, desire, and psychological exploration. They tap into primal instincts and societal narratives surrounding fertility, intimacy, and the very essence of human connection. Understanding the allure of breeding scenes requires a multifaceted approach that encompasses psychological, emotional, and cultural dimensions.

The Primal Instincts of Breeding

At the core of breeding scenes lies the primal instinct to procreate, a biological drive deeply embedded within our DNA. This drive is not merely about reproduction; it is intricately linked to the notions of legacy, survival, and the continuation of one's lineage. For many, the fantasy of breeding transcends the act itself, becoming a vehicle for exploring themes of dominance, submission, and vulnerability.

The psychological theory of *arousal transfer* posits that the heightened states of arousal associated with sexual activity can amplify feelings of intimacy and connection between partners. In breeding scenes, the act of engaging in a primal sexual encounter can evoke feelings of closeness and bonding, often leading to a deeper emotional connection.

Cultural Narratives and Societal Constructs

Breeding scenes also reflect and challenge cultural narratives surrounding sexuality and reproduction. In many societies, the act of breeding is laden with expectations and societal pressures, often idealized as the pinnacle of romantic relationships. Engaging in breeding scenes allows individuals to reclaim their narratives, empowering them to explore their desires without the constraints imposed by societal norms.

Moreover, breeding fantasies can serve as a counter-narrative to the often clinical and detached approach to sex and reproduction in modern society. By embracing breeding scenes, individuals can reconnect with the raw, visceral aspects of sexuality that are often sanitized in contemporary discourse.

Exploring Power Dynamics

Breeding scenes provide fertile ground for exploring power dynamics between partners. The interplay of dominance and submission can heighten the erotic charge of breeding scenarios, allowing participants to delve into their fantasies in a safe and consensual environment. This exploration can lead to a deeper understanding of one's own desires and boundaries, fostering personal growth and emotional intimacy.

For example, a submissive partner may find empowerment in surrendering control during a breeding scene, while a dominant partner may experience fulfillment in taking on the role of the initiator. This dynamic can create a powerful feedback loop, enhancing the overall experience for both parties involved.

The Importance of Communication and Consent

Engaging in breeding scenes necessitates a robust framework of communication and consent. Establishing clear boundaries and discussing desires openly is crucial to ensuring that all participants feel safe and respected. This dialogue not only enhances the experience but also fosters trust and intimacy, allowing individuals to explore their fantasies with confidence.

Incorporating elements such as safe words and aftercare practices can further enhance the emotional safety of breeding scenes. This attention to consent and communication transforms breeding from a mere physical act into a profound exploration of connection and vulnerability.

Personal Growth and Exploration

For many, breeding scenes are a pathway to personal growth and self-discovery. Engaging in such fantasies can help individuals confront their own beliefs and attitudes towards sexuality, reproduction, and intimacy. This exploration can lead to a more nuanced understanding of one's desires, ultimately enhancing one's sexual experiences and relationships.

Consider the example of a person who has long harbored fantasies of being part of a breeding scene but has felt societal pressure to suppress these desires. By embracing this aspect of their sexuality, they may find a newfound sense of liberation and empowerment, allowing them to fully inhabit their erotic identity.

Building Community and Connection

Finally, breeding scenes can foster a sense of community and connection among like-minded individuals. Engaging in these fantasies can create bonds that transcend traditional social constructs, allowing participants to connect over shared experiences and desires. This sense of belonging can be particularly valuable for those who may feel isolated or stigmatized in their sexual exploration.

In conclusion, breeding scenes offer a rich tapestry of experiences that encompass primal instincts, cultural narratives, power dynamics, and personal growth. By embracing these fantasies, individuals can explore their desires in a safe and consensual manner, ultimately enhancing their sexual experiences and deepening their connections with partners. The allure of breeding scenes lies not only in the act itself but also in the profound emotional and psychological journeys they inspire.

The Importance of Multiple Loads

The allure of multiple loads in breeding scenes transcends mere physical satisfaction; it taps into deeper psychological and emotional realms. Understanding the importance of multiple loads can enhance the breeding experience, fostering both intimacy and ecstasy. This section delves into the significance of multiple loads, exploring their psychological impact, the physiological aspects involved, and the ways in which they can elevate the erotic experience.

Psychological Impact of Multiple Loads

Multiple loads can serve as a powerful affirmation of sexual prowess and desirability. The act of experiencing multiple orgasms can create a sense of accomplishment and satisfaction, reinforcing self-esteem and body positivity. The psychological benefits are manifold:

- **Increased Confidence:** Successfully achieving multiple loads can boost confidence in one's sexual abilities, leading to a more fulfilling sexual experience.

- **Enhanced Intimacy:** Sharing the experience of multiple loads with a partner can deepen emotional bonds, creating a shared sense of vulnerability and trust.

- **Exploration of Fantasies:** Engaging in breeding scenes that emphasize multiple loads allows individuals to explore fantasies related to fertility, dominance, and submission, providing a safe space for sexual expression.

Physiological Aspects of Multiple Loads

From a physiological perspective, the ability to achieve multiple loads is tied to several factors, including arousal levels, hormonal responses, and the body's capacity for recovery between orgasms. The science behind multiple orgasms can be understood through the following concepts:

$$\text{Arousal Level} = f(\text{Physical Stimulation}, \text{Mental Engagement}) \quad (1)$$

Where:

- Physical Stimulation refers to the direct stimulation of erogenous zones.

- Mental Engagement encompasses fantasies, roleplay, and emotional connection.

The interplay between these factors can lead to heightened arousal, allowing for multiple ejaculation events. Additionally, the refractory period—the time following orgasm during which further orgasms are typically difficult to achieve—varies significantly among individuals. Factors influencing this include:

- **Age:** Younger individuals may experience shorter refractory periods, allowing for the potential of multiple loads.

- **Physical Health:** Overall fitness and health can enhance stamina and recovery time.

- **Mental State:** A relaxed and aroused mental state can reduce the refractory period, facilitating multiple orgasms.

Enhancing the Experience of Multiple Loads

To maximize the pleasure derived from multiple loads, certain techniques and practices can be employed:

- **Edging:** This technique involves bringing oneself or a partner close to orgasm and then stopping before climax. Repeating this process can lead to heightened intensity and the potential for multiple loads.

- **Prostate Stimulation:** For those with a prostate, incorporating prostate stimulation can lead to more intense orgasms and the possibility of multiple loads.

- **Variety of Techniques:** Utilizing different forms of stimulation—such as oral, manual, and penetrative—can keep arousal levels high and prolong the experience.

Common Challenges and Solutions

While the pursuit of multiple loads can be exhilarating, it may also come with challenges. Some common issues include:

- **Performance Anxiety:** The pressure to achieve multiple orgasms can lead to anxiety, detracting from the experience. To mitigate this, focus on the journey rather than the destination, allowing for organic pleasure to unfold.

- **Physical Discomfort:** Prolonged stimulation can lead to discomfort or overstimulation. Regular communication with partners about comfort levels and preferences is crucial.

- **Misalignment of Desires:** Partners may have differing expectations regarding the frequency and intensity of multiple loads. Open dialogue about desires and boundaries is essential to ensure a fulfilling experience for all involved.

Conclusion

In conclusion, the importance of multiple loads in breeding scenes lies not only in the physical pleasure they provide but also in the emotional and psychological benefits they offer. By understanding the interplay between arousal, physiological responses, and psychological factors, individuals can enhance their breeding experiences, forging deeper connections and exploring the full spectrum of their erotic desires. Embracing the journey towards multiple loads can lead to profound satisfaction and fulfillment, inviting participants to revel in the beauty of shared exploration and intimacy.

Fostering Deep Connections through Breeding

Breeding scenes can serve as a profound catalyst for intimacy and connection between partners. In this section, we will explore the psychological and emotional dimensions of breeding, emphasizing how these experiences can deepen relationships and foster a sense of belonging and trust.

The Psychological Underpinnings of Connection

At the core of human relationships lies the need for connection, which can be understood through various psychological theories. One relevant framework is **Attachment Theory**, which posits that the bonds formed in early childhood influence adult relationships. Secure attachments foster trust and intimacy, allowing individuals to explore their desires openly. In the context of breeding scenes, this secure base can encourage participants to engage in vulnerable behaviors, enhancing emotional closeness.

$$C = f(A, T, E) \qquad (2)$$

where C represents connection, A is attachment style, T is trust, and E is emotional expression. This equation illustrates that a strong connection (C) is a function of an individual's attachment style (A), the level of trust (T) established between partners, and the ability to express emotions (E) freely.

Building Trust Through Breeding Experiences

Trust is a cornerstone of any intimate relationship and is especially crucial in breeding scenes. Engaging in such intimate acts requires a high level of confidence in one's partner, as well as in the safety of the environment. Establishing trust can be achieved through:

- **Open Communication:** Discussing desires, boundaries, and fears prior to engaging in breeding can create a safe space. This dialogue should be ongoing, allowing partners to express their feelings and adjust their boundaries as needed.

- **Consistent Aftercare:** Aftercare is essential for reinforcing the bond between partners. It involves taking the time to reconnect emotionally after a scene, discussing what was enjoyable, and addressing any concerns. This practice not only enhances trust but also fosters a deeper emotional connection.

Creating Shared Experiences

Shared experiences can significantly enhance the connection between partners. Breeding scenes, when approached with mutual consent and enthusiasm, can create powerful memories that bind individuals together. Engaging in these experiences allows partners to explore their fantasies collectively, which can lead to increased satisfaction and emotional intimacy.

For example, consider a couple that decides to incorporate roleplay into their breeding scene. By adopting different personas, they can explore various dynamics and desires, leading to a richer experience. This shared exploration can create a sense of unity and understanding, as both partners navigate their fantasies together.

Navigating Challenges in Breeding Scenes

Despite the potential for deep connections, breeding scenes can also present challenges that may hinder emotional bonding. Common issues include:

- **Miscommunication:** Misunderstandings about boundaries or desires can lead to discomfort or emotional distress. Clear communication before and during the scene is essential to mitigate these risks.

- **Emotional Vulnerability:** Engaging in breeding can evoke strong emotions, including fear or anxiety. It is crucial for partners to recognize these feelings and provide support to one another.

Addressing these challenges involves ongoing dialogue and a commitment to understanding each partner's emotional landscape. Regular check-ins can help partners navigate their feelings and reinforce their connection.

The Role of Aftercare in Fostering Connection

Aftercare is a critical component of breeding scenes that can significantly enhance emotional connection. This practice involves nurturing one another after an intense experience, allowing partners to process their feelings and reaffirm their bond. Effective aftercare can include:

- **Physical Comfort:** Cuddling, gentle touches, or providing a warm blanket can create a sense of safety and intimacy.

- **Verbal Reassurance:** Sharing affirmations about the experience can help partners feel valued and understood. Phrases like "I loved that we explored this together" can reinforce the positive aspects of the encounter.

Incorporating aftercare into breeding scenes not only aids in emotional recovery but also strengthens the relational foundation, allowing partners to feel more connected and secure.

Conclusion

Fostering deep connections through breeding is a multifaceted process that involves trust, communication, shared experiences, and effective aftercare. By understanding the psychological underpinnings of intimacy and addressing potential challenges, partners can create a nurturing environment that enhances their emotional bond. Engaging in breeding scenes with a focus on connection can lead to profound transformations in relationships, allowing individuals to explore their desires while deepening their love and trust for one another.

Ultimately, the journey of fostering connection through breeding is an ongoing one, requiring commitment, empathy, and a willingness to explore the depths of intimacy together.

How This Guide Will Enhance Your Breeding Experience

In the realm of erotic exploration, breeding scenes stand out as a unique and deeply intimate experience that can foster connections between partners. This guide is designed to enhance your breeding experience in several profound ways, ensuring that every encounter is not only pleasurable but also safe, consensual, and fulfilling.

1. Empowering Knowledge

Knowledge is power, especially in the context of breeding scenes. By understanding the intricacies of male anatomy, the science behind multiple orgasms, and the psychological aspects of breeding, you can navigate these experiences with confidence. For instance, familiarizing yourself with the concept of *multiple orgasms* can significantly enhance your ability to prolong pleasure. The physiological basis can be expressed through the following equation, which illustrates the relationship between arousal and orgasm:

$$P = \frac{A}{R} \qquad (3)$$

where P is the pleasure experienced, A is the level of arousal, and R is the resistance to orgasm. By increasing arousal and managing resistance through techniques such as edging, you can create a cycle of pleasure that leads to multiple loads, enriching the breeding experience.

2. Enhanced Communication Skills

Effective communication is the cornerstone of any successful breeding scene. This guide emphasizes the importance of establishing clear boundaries, safe words, and mutual expectations. Through practical exercises and negotiation techniques outlined in this guide, you will learn how to articulate your desires and listen to your partner's needs. For example, engaging in a pre-scene negotiation session can set the stage for a more satisfying encounter. Consider the following structure for a negotiation:

- Discuss individual desires and fantasies.
- Establish hard and soft limits.
- Agree on safe words and signals.
- Review health and safety considerations.

By fostering an environment of open dialogue, you can build trust and intimacy, which are essential for a fulfilling breeding experience.

3. Creating the Ideal Environment

The ambiance of your breeding space plays a crucial role in the overall experience. This guide provides insights into setting the scene with sensory elements that stimulate arousal, such as lighting, scents, and sounds. For example, the use of dim lighting can create a sense of intimacy, while specific scents can enhance relaxation and desire. Consider incorporating elements such as:

- Soft music to create a sensual atmosphere.
- Aromatherapy with essential oils like jasmine or sandalwood to enhance relaxation.
- Comfortable bedding and props that encourage exploration and play.

By thoughtfully designing your breeding environment, you can elevate the experience, making it more immersive and pleasurable.

4. Techniques for Maximizing Pleasure

This guide delves into various techniques that can amplify pleasure during breeding scenes. From foreplay and teasing to incorporating roleplay and fantasy, you will discover methods to heighten anticipation and intensify orgasms. For example, employing *dirty talk* can significantly enhance arousal, as it taps into the psychological aspects of desire. Research suggests that verbal stimulation can activate the same pleasure centers in the brain as physical touch.

Additionally, exploring prostate stimulation can unlock new levels of pleasure for male participants. Understanding the anatomy and employing the right techniques can lead to powerful orgasms and a richer breeding experience.

5. Safety and Consent as Foundations

Safety and consent are paramount in breeding scenes. This guide emphasizes the need to establish and maintain consent throughout your encounters. By understanding the nuances of consent, including verbal and non-verbal signals, you can create a safe space for exploration. The following principles can guide you:

- Always seek enthusiastic consent.
- Be aware of and respect your partner's boundaries.
- Continuously check in during the scene to ensure comfort and enjoyment.

By prioritizing safety and consent, you can create a nurturing environment that allows for deeper exploration and connection.

6. Emotional and Mental Well-being

Engaging in breeding scenes can evoke a range of emotions. This guide addresses the importance of processing these feelings through aftercare and debriefing. Aftercare is a vital component that allows partners to reconnect and address any emotional challenges that may arise. Techniques for effective aftercare include:

- Engaging in cuddling or physical touch to foster connection.
- Discussing the scene to process feelings and experiences.
- Practicing self-care to address any emotional needs.

By incorporating these practices, you can enhance emotional well-being and strengthen the bond between partners.

Conclusion

In summary, this guide is a comprehensive resource that will enhance your breeding experience by empowering you with knowledge, improving communication, creating the ideal environment, maximizing pleasure, ensuring safety and consent, and addressing emotional well-being. By embracing the principles and techniques outlined herein, you will embark on a journey of erotic exploration that is both fulfilling and transformative. Whether you are a novice or an experienced participant in breeding scenes, this guide offers valuable insights that will enrich your encounters and foster deeper connections.

Understanding Breeding Scenes

Defining Breeding Scenes

Exploring Different Types of Breeding

Breeding scenes encompass a rich tapestry of desires and fantasies that can manifest in various forms. Understanding these different types is crucial for anyone looking to delve deeper into the breeding lifestyle. This section will explore the nuances of breeding dynamics, providing insights into the motivations, experiences, and contexts that define them.

1. Traditional Breeding

Traditional breeding typically refers to the act of unprotected intercourse with the intent of conception. This type of breeding scene is often steeped in cultural and personal significance, as it may evoke feelings of intimacy, trust, and a primal connection. Participants may engage in this practice for a variety of reasons, including:

- **Desire for Parenthood:** Many individuals and couples find the idea of creating life to be a deeply fulfilling experience. The act of breeding becomes intertwined with their hopes and dreams for a family.

- **Intimacy and Bonding:** The physical act of breeding can enhance emotional connections, allowing partners to explore vulnerability and trust in a profound way.

- **Cultural or Religious Significance:** In some cultures, breeding is viewed as a sacred duty, and engaging in this act can carry significant weight within the community.

2. Fantasy Breeding

Fantasy breeding, on the other hand, is characterized by the exploration of breeding themes without the actual intent or possibility of conception. This type of breeding scene can take many forms, including role-play scenarios, where participants may embody characters that heighten the eroticism of the act. Key aspects include:

- **Role-Playing:** Participants may adopt roles such as a dominant "breeder" and a submissive "breeding mare," creating a power dynamic that enhances the experience.

- **Safe Exploration:** Fantasy breeding allows individuals to engage in breeding themes without the associated risks of pregnancy or sexually transmitted infections (STIs). This can create a safe space for exploring desires.

- **Creative Scenarios:** Couples may craft elaborate narratives, incorporating elements of taboo or forbidden desires, which can amplify arousal and excitement.

3. Group Breeding

Group breeding scenes involve multiple participants and can range from threesomes to larger orgies. These scenes can bring a heightened sense of excitement and community, as well as present unique challenges. Considerations include:

- **Dynamics of Consent:** In group settings, clear communication and consent become paramount. Establishing boundaries and ensuring everyone is comfortable with the scene is essential.

- **Health and Safety:** The risks of STIs increase in group settings, necessitating discussions about protection and sexual health. Participants should agree on safety protocols before engaging.

- **Emotional Considerations:** Group breeding can evoke feelings of jealousy or insecurity among participants. Open dialogue before and after the scene can help mitigate these feelings.

4. Public Breeding

Public breeding scenes take the concept of breeding into shared or semi-public spaces. These scenarios can heighten the thrill of being caught or observed, appealing to those who enjoy exhibitionism. Important factors include:

- **Legal and Ethical Considerations:** Engaging in public breeding requires an understanding of local laws and the ethics of consent, particularly regarding bystanders who may not consent to being part of the scene.

- **Negotiating Boundaries:** Participants must discuss and agree on what is acceptable in a public setting, including the level of exposure and interaction with onlookers.

- **Building Community:** Public breeding can foster a sense of belonging and community among participants, as they share in the excitement of the experience together.

5. Solo Breeding

While breeding is often thought of as a shared experience, solo breeding allows individuals to explore their desires independently. This practice can include self-stimulation with the intent of embodying the breeding fantasy. Aspects to consider include:

- **Self-Exploration:** Solo breeding can serve as a means of self-discovery, allowing individuals to understand their own desires and fantasies without the influence of a partner.

- **Role Development:** Individuals can create narratives and characters for themselves, embodying the roles they desire to explore in a safe and private setting.

- **Toys and Accessories:** The use of sex toys can enhance the solo breeding experience, providing additional stimulation and facilitating the exploration of different sensations.

6. Theoretical Considerations

From a psychological perspective, breeding scenes can be analyzed through various lenses, including:

- **Attachment Theory:** The desire for breeding may be linked to attachment styles, where individuals seek to create bonds through physical intimacy.

- **Erotic Fantasy:** Breeding can serve as a powerful erotic fantasy that taps into primal instincts and societal taboos, leading to heightened arousal.

- **Social Dynamics:** The interplay of power, consent, and emotional connection in breeding scenes reflects broader societal norms and individual desires.

In conclusion, exploring the different types of breeding allows individuals to understand their desires more fully and engage in experiences that resonate with their fantasies. Whether through traditional, fantasy, group, public, or solo breeding, the key is to prioritize communication, consent, and safety, ensuring that all participants can enjoy fulfilling and pleasurable experiences.

The Psychology of Breeding Scenes

Breeding scenes tap into deep-seated psychological desires and fantasies, often intertwining elements of power, intimacy, and primal instincts. Understanding the psychology behind these scenes can enhance the experience for all participants, fostering a deeper connection and mutual satisfaction.

The Role of Fantasy

At the core of breeding scenes lies the element of fantasy. Many individuals are drawn to the idea of breeding due to its association with fertility, creation, and the primal urge to procreate. This fantasy can be rooted in various psychological theories, including Freud's concept of the libido, which posits that sexual desire is a fundamental driving force in human behavior. Breeding fantasies often evoke feelings of safety, security, and belonging, as they can symbolize a deeper connection between partners.

Attachment Theory

Attachment theory, developed by John Bowlby, provides insight into how individuals form emotional bonds and connections. In breeding scenes, participants may experience heightened feelings of attachment and intimacy. The act of engaging in a breeding scene can trigger the release of oxytocin, often referred to as the "love hormone," which is associated with bonding and trust. This hormonal response can lead to a stronger emotional connection, enhancing the overall experience.

DEFINING BREEDING SCENES

Power Dynamics and Control

Breeding scenes often incorporate elements of power dynamics, which can evoke feelings of dominance and submission. The psychological thrill of surrendering control or taking charge can be exhilarating for participants. According to the BDSM community, the negotiation of power dynamics is crucial for establishing consent and ensuring a safe environment. Participants may find fulfillment in exploring their roles, whether as a dominant "breeder" or a submissive "breeder," allowing them to express their desires and fantasies.

The Primal Instincts

Breeding taps into primal instincts that are hardwired into human psychology. The desire to reproduce is a fundamental aspect of human nature, and breeding scenes can evoke feelings of raw, animalistic passion. This primal urge can be both exhilarating and terrifying, as it confronts individuals with their most basic instincts. The psychological interplay between fear and desire can heighten arousal, creating a potent mix of emotions that enhances the breeding experience.

Potential Psychological Challenges

While breeding scenes can be fulfilling, they may also present psychological challenges. Participants must navigate complex emotions, including jealousy, insecurity, and fear of judgment. It is essential to address these feelings openly and honestly through communication and negotiation. Establishing boundaries and safe words can help mitigate potential issues, ensuring that all participants feel secure and respected throughout the experience.

Case Study: A Breeding Scene Experience

To illustrate the psychological dynamics at play in breeding scenes, consider the following hypothetical scenario:
    Scenario: Sarah and Jake have been exploring their breeding fantasies together. After establishing clear boundaries and discussing their desires, they decide to engage in a breeding scene. Sarah takes on the submissive role, while Jake embraces his dominant instincts. As they progress, Sarah feels a rush of excitement and vulnerability, surrendering control to Jake. This dynamic enhances their emotional connection, allowing them to explore deeper levels of intimacy.

Throughout the scene, they communicate openly, checking in with each other to ensure comfort and consent. The experience culminates in a heightened sense of pleasure and connection, reinforcing their bond and fulfilling their desires.

Conclusion

Understanding the psychology of breeding scenes is crucial for creating a fulfilling and enjoyable experience. By exploring fantasies, navigating power dynamics, and addressing potential psychological challenges, participants can foster deeper connections and enhance their breeding experiences. Ultimately, the psychological interplay of desire, attachment, and primal instincts makes breeding scenes a rich and rewarding aspect of erotic exploration.

The Role of Consent in Breeding Scenes

Consent is a foundational element in any sexual encounter, particularly in the context of breeding scenes, where the stakes may feel higher due to the emotional and physical implications involved. Understanding the nuances of consent not only enhances the experience but also fosters trust and safety among participants. This section delves into the various dimensions of consent, its importance, and practical applications within breeding scenarios.

Defining Consent

Consent is defined as an agreement between participants to engage in specific sexual activities. It is essential that this agreement is informed, enthusiastic, and revocable at any time. In the context of breeding scenes, consent takes on additional layers, as participants may have varying desires and boundaries regarding intimacy, vulnerability, and the implications of potential pregnancy.

The Importance of Informed Consent

Informed consent requires that all parties have a clear understanding of what they are agreeing to. In breeding scenes, this encompasses discussions about:

- **Intentions:** Are all participants aware of the potential outcomes of breeding, including emotional attachment and the possibility of conception?

- **Health and Safety:** Are participants aware of each other's sexual health status? This includes discussions about STIs, pregnancy prevention, and any relevant medical histories.

- **Expectations:** What does each participant hope to gain from the experience? Open dialogue about desires and fantasies can help align expectations and enhance satisfaction.

Enthusiastic Consent

Enthusiastic consent goes beyond mere agreement; it embodies a genuine desire to participate. In breeding scenes, this can manifest through verbal affirmations, body language, and ongoing communication throughout the encounter. Participants should feel empowered to express their enthusiasm or lack thereof at any moment.

$$\text{Enthusiastic Consent} = \text{Desire} + \text{Willingness} + \text{Communication} \quad (4)$$

This equation highlights the interplay between desire, willingness, and communication in achieving enthusiastic consent. Each component must be present for consent to be truly valid.

Revocability of Consent

One of the most critical aspects of consent is its revocability. Participants must understand that consent can be withdrawn at any time, and this withdrawal must be respected immediately. This is particularly important in breeding scenes, where emotional and physical states can shift rapidly.

$$\text{Revocable Consent} \Rightarrow \text{Immediate Respect for Boundaries} \quad (5)$$

This principle emphasizes that once consent is revoked, all participants must honor the new boundaries without question or hesitation.

Consent Signals

Understanding and recognizing consent signals is crucial in breeding scenes. These signals can be verbal or non-verbal and must be monitored continuously.

- **Verbal Signals:** Clear and affirmative statements such as "yes," "I want this," or "please continue" signify consent.

- **Non-Verbal Signals:** Body language, facial expressions, and physical responsiveness can indicate consent or discomfort. For instance, leaning in closer may suggest eagerness, while pulling away may indicate a need for pause or reconsideration.

Navigating Emotional Boundaries

Breeding scenes can evoke strong emotions, including vulnerability, intimacy, and attachment. Participants should engage in discussions about emotional boundaries prior to the encounter. This includes:

- **Aftercare Needs:** Understanding what each participant requires post-scene to feel safe and supported.

- **Potential Emotional Outcomes:** Discussing how participants may feel during and after the scene, and how to handle unexpected emotions.

Consent in Group Breeding Dynamics

When multiple participants are involved, establishing consent becomes even more complex. It is vital to ensure that each person's boundaries are respected and that all participants are comfortable with the dynamics at play.

- **Group Agreements:** Establish clear agreements about what activities are permissible and ensure that everyone is on the same page.

- **Ongoing Check-Ins:** Regularly check in with each participant to gauge comfort levels and adjust activities as necessary.

Consent in Public Breeding Scenes

Public breeding scenes introduce additional layers of complexity regarding consent. Participants must navigate not only their own boundaries but also the potential for onlookers and the legal implications of public displays of sexuality.

- **Privacy Considerations:** Discuss how much privacy is expected and what measures will be taken to maintain it.

- **Legal Boundaries:** Be aware of the laws governing public sexual activity in your jurisdiction to avoid legal repercussions.

Conclusion

In summary, consent is a multifaceted and dynamic aspect of breeding scenes that requires ongoing communication, respect, and understanding. By prioritizing informed, enthusiastic, and revocable consent, participants can create a safe and pleasurable environment that enhances their breeding experiences. This commitment to consent not only fosters trust and intimacy but also empowers individuals to explore their desires within a framework of safety and respect.

Breaking Down Stereotypes and Misconceptions about Breeding

Breeding scenes, often shrouded in taboo and misunderstanding, can evoke a plethora of reactions ranging from intrigue to aversion. To fully embrace the breeding lifestyle, it is essential to dismantle the stereotypes and misconceptions that surround it. This section aims to clarify common misunderstandings and provide a nuanced perspective on the dynamics of breeding scenes.

1. The Myth of Objectification

One prevalent stereotype is that breeding reduces individuals to mere vessels for procreation, stripping away their autonomy and identity. This misconception overlooks the fundamental principles of consent and mutual desire that underpin breeding scenes. In reality, breeding is often a deeply intimate experience that fosters connection between partners. It is crucial to recognize that participants engage in breeding willingly and enthusiastically, with a shared understanding of their roles.

To illustrate, consider a couple who engages in breeding as an expression of their love and trust. They communicate openly about their desires, boundaries, and intentions, creating a safe space where both partners can explore their fantasies without fear of judgment or coercion. This dynamic exemplifies how breeding can enhance intimacy rather than diminish individuality.

2. The Fallacy of Gender Roles

Another common misconception is the rigid adherence to traditional gender roles within breeding scenes. Many believe that breeding is solely a heterosexual activity, where men are dominant and women are submissive. This stereotype fails to account for the diverse range of sexual orientations and relationship dynamics that exist in contemporary society.

Breeding scenes can be inclusive of all genders and sexual identities. For instance, a polyamorous group may engage in breeding activities that challenge conventional norms, allowing for a fluid exchange of roles and power dynamics. In such scenarios, participants can explore their desires in a manner that transcends traditional gender expectations, fostering a more inclusive and enriching experience.

3. The Misunderstanding of Safety and Health

A significant misconception surrounding breeding is the belief that it inherently poses health risks and lacks safety protocols. While it is true that breeding can involve the exchange of bodily fluids, responsible participants prioritize health and safety through clear communication and established practices.

For example, couples can engage in pre-breeding discussions about sexual health, including STI testing and contraception options. By addressing these concerns openly, partners can mitigate risks while enjoying their breeding experiences. Furthermore, the use of safe words and negotiation techniques ensures that all parties feel secure and respected throughout the encounter.

4. The Stigma of Public Breeding

Public breeding scenes often attract scrutiny and stigma, with many perceiving them as inappropriate or immoral. This perspective fails to acknowledge the consensual nature of such encounters and the thrill that can accompany them. Public breeding can be a form of expression that allows participants to explore their sexuality in a shared space, fostering community and connection among like-minded individuals.

Consider a gathering where individuals openly engage in breeding activities. Participants may feel liberated by the shared experience, creating an atmosphere of acceptance and exploration. When conducted with consent and respect for boundaries, public breeding can contribute to a vibrant and supportive community.

5. The Misconception of Breeding as a Solely Physical Act

Many individuals mistakenly view breeding as purely a physical act, neglecting the emotional and psychological dimensions involved. Breeding can evoke powerful feelings of intimacy, vulnerability, and connection, transcending the mere act of intercourse.

For instance, the act of breeding can symbolize a deep commitment between partners, reinforcing their bond and shared desires. Engaging in breeding scenes can facilitate emotional growth and deeper connections, allowing participants to explore their fantasies within a safe and trusting environment.

Conclusion

Breaking down stereotypes and misconceptions about breeding is essential for fostering a more inclusive and understanding community. By recognizing the complexities of breeding scenes, individuals can embrace their desires without fear of judgment. Through open communication, consent, and a commitment to safety, breeding can be a fulfilling and enriching aspect of one's erotic lifestyle. As society continues to evolve, it is crucial to challenge outdated beliefs and celebrate the diversity of experiences that breeding has to offer.

Preparing for Breeding Scenes

Communication and Negotiation

Establishing Boundaries and Safe Words

In the realm of breeding scenes, establishing boundaries and safe words is paramount for ensuring a consensual and pleasurable experience. This process not only fosters a sense of safety but also enhances the overall intimacy between partners. Understanding the significance of boundaries and safe words can transform a breeding experience from a mere physical encounter into a deeply connected exploration of desires and fantasies.

The Importance of Boundaries

Boundaries serve as the framework within which all participants can explore their desires without fear of crossing into uncomfortable or unwanted territory. They delineate what is acceptable and what is not, allowing individuals to express their needs and limits openly. In the context of breeding scenes, boundaries may encompass various aspects, including:

- **Physical Boundaries:** These refer to the types of physical activities that are permissible. For example, one partner may be comfortable with oral stimulation but not with penetration.

- **Emotional Boundaries:** These involve the emotional aspects of the scene, such as the level of intimacy or vulnerability that each partner is willing to share.

- **Time Boundaries:** Establishing how long the scene will last can help manage expectations and ensure that all participants feel comfortable throughout the experience.

- **Health and Safety Boundaries:** This includes discussions about contraception, sexually transmitted infections (STIs), and any health-related concerns that may arise during the scene.

Communicating Boundaries

Effective communication is the cornerstone of establishing boundaries. Partners should engage in open and honest discussions about their desires, limits, and any past experiences that may influence their current preferences. This dialogue can take place in a relaxed setting, allowing both parties to feel at ease as they share their thoughts.

A practical approach to discussing boundaries includes the following steps:

1. **Create a Safe Space:** Choose a comfortable environment where both partners can speak freely without distractions.

2. **Use "I" Statements:** Encourage each partner to express their feelings using "I" statements, such as "I feel comfortable with…" or "I would prefer to avoid…". This reduces the likelihood of defensiveness and promotes understanding.

3. **Listen Actively:** Each partner should practice active listening, ensuring that they fully understand the other's boundaries before proceeding.

4. **Document Boundaries:** Consider writing down agreed-upon boundaries and safe words to refer back to if needed.

Choosing Safe Words

Safe words are a crucial component of any erotic scene, acting as a signal to pause or stop the activity if one partner feels uncomfortable or overwhelmed. The effectiveness of a safe word lies in its clarity and memorability. Here are some guidelines for selecting safe words:

- **Simplicity:** Choose a word that is easy to remember and pronounce, even in the heat of the moment. Common choices include "red" for stop and "yellow" for slow down.

- **Uniqueness:** Select a word that is unlikely to come up in regular conversation during the scene. This ensures that it will stand out as a clear signal.

- **Agreement:** Both partners must agree on the safe word and understand its meaning. This mutual understanding reinforces trust and safety.

Addressing Potential Problems

While establishing boundaries and safe words is essential, challenges may arise. Some common issues include:

- **Miscommunication:** Partners may misinterpret each other's boundaries. To mitigate this, regular check-ins during the scene can help clarify any uncertainties.

- **Overstepping Boundaries:** Sometimes, one partner may forget or disregard established boundaries in the heat of the moment. This highlights the importance of having a safe word readily available.

- **Emotional Responses:** Breeding scenes can evoke strong emotions. If one partner feels overwhelmed, it is vital to respect their safe word and pause the scene for a debriefing.

Examples of Effective Communication

To illustrate the process of establishing boundaries and safe words, consider the following example:

Amber and Jake sit down for a pre-scene discussion. Amber expresses her desire to explore breeding but shares her concern about the intensity of the experience. They agree on a safe word, "pineapple," to use if either feels uncomfortable. They also discuss their physical boundaries, deciding that Amber is open to oral stimulation and penetration, but only if they use protection. Jake reassures Amber that her comfort is his priority, and they agree to check in with each other throughout the scene.

In conclusion, establishing boundaries and safe words is a vital step in preparing for breeding scenes. By fostering open communication and mutual respect, partners can create a safe and pleasurable environment that enhances their connection and exploration of desires. Emphasizing the importance of boundaries and safe words not only protects participants but also deepens the intimacy and trust that are essential for a fulfilling breeding experience.

Discussing Expectations and Desires

In the realm of breeding scenes, discussing expectations and desires is a fundamental step that sets the stage for a mutually satisfying experience. Open dialogue not only fosters intimacy but also establishes a framework of trust and safety that is crucial for exploring such intimate dynamics. This section will explore the theory behind effective communication, common problems that may arise, and practical examples to guide you through this essential aspect of your breeding journey.

Theoretical Framework

Effective communication is grounded in several key theories, including the *Social Exchange Theory* and the *Communication Privacy Management Theory*. The Social Exchange Theory posits that relationships are built on the exchange of resources, which can include emotional support, intimacy, and sexual satisfaction. In breeding scenes, participants must openly discuss what they hope to gain and what they are willing to offer, creating a balance that satisfies both parties.

Communication Privacy Management Theory emphasizes the importance of boundaries in sharing personal information. In breeding scenes, where desires can be deeply personal and sometimes taboo, it is vital to establish what is shared and what remains private. This approach allows individuals to feel safe in expressing their desires without fear of judgment or breach of confidentiality.

Common Problems

Despite the importance of discussing expectations, several common problems can arise during these conversations:

- **Miscommunication:** Misunderstandings can lead to unmet expectations. For example, one partner may assume that the other desires a specific type of breeding scene, while the other may have different preferences.

- **Fear of Vulnerability:** Discussing desires can make individuals feel exposed. The fear of rejection or ridicule may prevent honest communication, leading to frustration and disappointment.

- **Power Imbalances:** In some dynamics, one partner may dominate the conversation, leaving the other feeling unheard. This imbalance can create resentment and hinder the development of a fulfilling breeding experience.

COMMUNICATION AND NEGOTIATION

Practical Examples

To navigate these challenges effectively, consider the following practical examples and techniques:

1. Use Open-Ended Questions Encourage dialogue by asking open-ended questions that invite detailed responses. For instance:

> "What aspects of breeding excite you the most, and why?"

This question not only invites the partner to share their desires but also opens the floor for a deeper discussion about their motivations.

2. Establish a Safe Space Create an environment conducive to open dialogue. This could be a quiet, comfortable setting where both partners feel relaxed. For example, consider initiating the conversation during a cozy evening at home, perhaps over a glass of wine, where both partners can speak freely without distractions.

3. Utilize Active Listening Techniques Practice active listening by reflecting back what your partner has shared. For instance:

> "It sounds like you really enjoy the idea of multiple partners in a breeding scene. Can you tell me more about what that means for you?"

This technique not only validates your partner's feelings but also encourages them to elaborate on their desires.

4. Set Clear Boundaries Discuss and agree upon boundaries before engaging in breeding scenes. For example, if one partner desires to explore public breeding while the other prefers private settings, acknowledging these boundaries early on can prevent discomfort later.

5. Create a Desire List Consider creating a list of desires and expectations together. This could include preferences for specific activities, the number of participants, or desired emotional connections. By visualizing these desires, both partners can gain clarity and alignment on their breeding goals.

Conclusion

Discussing expectations and desires is not merely a preliminary step; it is an ongoing dialogue that evolves as partners explore their breeding lifestyle together. By employing effective communication strategies, recognizing potential problems, and utilizing practical techniques, individuals can create a nurturing environment where their breeding experiences can flourish. Remember, the journey of exploration is as important as the destination, and through open dialogue, you can cultivate a deeper connection with your partner, ultimately enhancing your breeding experience.

Addressing Health and Safety Concerns

In the realm of breeding scenes, ensuring health and safety is paramount. Engaging in intimate activities carries inherent risks, and being well-informed is crucial for a fulfilling and safe experience. This section will explore various health and safety concerns, offer practical solutions, and emphasize the importance of communication and consent.

Understanding Health Risks

Engaging in breeding scenes can expose participants to several health risks, including sexually transmitted infections (STIs) and unintended pregnancies. It is essential to understand these risks to make informed choices. The primary health concerns include:

- **Sexually Transmitted Infections (STIs):** STIs can be transmitted through unprotected sexual contact. Common STIs include chlamydia, gonorrhea, syphilis, herpes, and HIV. The risk of transmission increases with multiple partners or lack of protection.

- **Unintended Pregnancies:** Breeding scenes often revolve around the fantasy of conception. However, it is crucial to discuss and understand the implications of potential pregnancies. Participants should consider their reproductive choices and use appropriate contraception if pregnancy is not desired.

Preventative Measures

To mitigate health risks, participants should adopt several preventative measures:

- **Regular STI Testing:** Regular testing for STIs is essential for sexually active individuals. Both partners should discuss their testing history and ensure they are up to date with screenings. The Centers for Disease Control and Prevention (CDC) recommends testing at least once a year for sexually active individuals, especially those with multiple partners.

- **Contraceptive Options:** Discussing contraceptive methods is vital in breeding scenes. Options include hormonal methods (e.g., pills, patches, IUDs), barrier methods (e.g., condoms, dental dams), and fertility awareness methods. Each method has its effectiveness rate, which can be calculated using the following equation:

$$\text{Effectiveness Rate} = \frac{\text{Number of pregnancies prevented}}{\text{Total number of couples using the method}} \times 100 \tag{6}$$

- **Safe Practices:** Using barrier methods, such as condoms, can significantly reduce the risk of STIs and unintended pregnancies. It is important to ensure that barriers are used correctly and consistently throughout the scene.

Communication and Consent

Open communication about health and safety concerns is essential in breeding scenes. Participants should engage in discussions about their sexual health, boundaries, and expectations. This dialogue fosters trust and intimacy, making the experience more enjoyable.

- **Sharing Health Histories:** Partners should feel comfortable sharing their sexual health histories, including any STIs, previous partners, and contraceptive use. This transparency helps build a foundation of trust and allows for informed decision-making.

- **Discussing Boundaries:** Establishing clear boundaries regarding health and safety is crucial. Participants should communicate their limits regarding sexual practices, including preferences for protection and comfort levels with certain activities.

- **Establishing Safe Words:** Implementing safe words can help participants navigate their experiences safely. A safe word allows individuals to pause or stop the activity if they feel uncomfortable or unsafe.

Aftercare and Emotional Well-being

Aftercare is an essential component of any intimate scene, particularly in breeding scenarios. Participants should take time to reconnect and discuss their experiences. This practice not only addresses any physical discomfort but also fosters emotional well-being.

- **Debriefing:** Aftercare should include a debriefing session where partners can share their feelings and thoughts about the experience. This process helps address any concerns and reinforces emotional intimacy.

- **Physical Comfort:** Providing physical comfort, such as cuddling or gentle touch, can help ease any tension and enhance emotional connection.

- **Emotional Check-ins:** Participants should check in with each other regarding their emotional state post-scene. This practice ensures that both partners feel supported and validated in their feelings.

Conclusion

Addressing health and safety concerns in breeding scenes is essential for a fulfilling and enjoyable experience. By understanding potential risks, implementing preventative measures, and fostering open communication, participants can create a safe and intimate environment. Remember, the key to a successful breeding scene lies in mutual respect, consent, and a commitment to each other's well-being. Embrace the journey, and prioritize health and safety as you explore the depths of your desires.

Building Trust and Intimacy through Open Communication

In the realm of breeding scenes, the foundation of trust and intimacy is paramount. Open communication serves as the bedrock upon which fulfilling and consensual experiences are built. This section explores the theories and practical approaches that underscore the importance of dialogue in fostering deep connections between partners.

Theoretical Framework

Open communication can be understood through the lens of several psychological theories, notably the **Communication Privacy Management Theory (CPM)** and the **Attachment Theory**.

Communication Privacy Management Theory posits that individuals maintain boundaries around private information and negotiate those boundaries with others. In the context of breeding scenes, this theory highlights the necessity for partners to discuss their desires, limits, and expectations clearly. Misunderstandings can lead to discomfort or even harm, making it essential to articulate personal boundaries effectively.

Attachment Theory, on the other hand, emphasizes the role of early relationships in shaping our ability to form close bonds. Secure attachment styles promote open communication, while anxious or avoidant styles may hinder it. Recognizing one's attachment style can be beneficial in navigating conversations about breeding, as it allows individuals to understand their own needs and how they may affect their partner's comfort levels.

Common Problems in Communication

Despite the importance of open dialogue, several barriers can impede effective communication in breeding scenes:

1. **Fear of Judgment:** Partners may hesitate to express their desires or limits due to fear of being judged or misunderstood. This fear can stifle honest conversation and lead to resentment or unmet needs.

2. **Assumptions and Misinterpretations:** Assuming that one partner knows what the other wants can lead to miscommunication. Each individual has unique preferences and boundaries, and failing to clarify these can result in negative experiences.

3. **Emotional Vulnerability:** Discussing intimate desires can evoke feelings of vulnerability. Partners may struggle to articulate their needs, fearing that doing so could jeopardize the relationship or the scene itself.

4. **Inconsistent Communication:** Communication should be ongoing. Relying on a single conversation to cover all bases can lead to misunderstandings later on. Partners must remain open to revisiting discussions as their desires and boundaries evolve.

Strategies for Effective Communication

To overcome these barriers, consider the following strategies:

- **Create a Safe Space:** Establish an environment where both partners feel comfortable expressing themselves. This can be achieved by choosing a neutral location, minimizing distractions, and ensuring that both parties are in a relaxed state of mind.

- **Use "I" Statements:** Frame your thoughts using "I" statements to express feelings without placing blame. For example, "I feel anxious when we don't discuss our boundaries" is more constructive than "You never talk about limits."

- **Active Listening:** Practice active listening by giving full attention to your partner when they speak. Reflect back what you hear to ensure understanding. This not only shows respect but also fosters deeper intimacy.

- **Set Aside Time for Conversations:** Designate specific times for discussions about desires and boundaries, separate from the actual breeding scenes. This helps to ensure that both partners can focus on the conversation without the pressure of immediate sexual context.

- **Check-In Regularly:** Make it a habit to check in with each other before, during, and after breeding scenes. This can be as simple as asking, "How are you feeling?" or "Is there anything you'd like to adjust?" These check-ins reinforce trust and demonstrate care for each other's well-being.

Examples of Open Communication in Breeding Scenes

To illustrate the power of open communication, consider the following scenarios:

> **Example**
>
> **Scenario 1: Setting Boundaries**
> Before engaging in a breeding scene, partners may discuss their limits. For instance, one partner might express, "I'm comfortable with vaginal intercourse but not anal." This clear communication establishes boundaries that both partners can respect, creating a safer and more enjoyable experience.
>
> **Scenario 2: Expressing Desires**
> During a breeding scene, one partner may feel the urge to explore a new fantasy. They might say, "I'd love to try roleplaying as a doctor and patient." This open expression of desire allows the other partner to respond positively or set limits, enhancing the overall experience through mutual consent and understanding.

Conclusion

Building trust and intimacy through open communication is essential for successful breeding scenes. By understanding the theoretical frameworks that support effective dialogue, recognizing common problems, and implementing practical strategies, partners can create a safe and fulfilling environment for exploration. Ultimately, the journey into breeding is not just about physical pleasure; it is an opportunity to deepen emotional connections and foster lasting trust. As you embark on this adventure, remember that every conversation is a step toward a more profound intimacy and understanding of one another.

Dynamic Negotiation Techniques for Successful Breeding Scenes

Negotiation is a crucial aspect of any intimate encounter, particularly in the context of breeding scenes where desires, boundaries, and emotional investments intersect. Dynamic negotiation techniques provide a framework for ensuring that all participants feel safe, respected, and fulfilled. This section outlines effective strategies for negotiating breeding scenes, emphasizing the importance of communication, flexibility, and emotional awareness.

Understanding Dynamic Negotiation

Dynamic negotiation is an ongoing process that adapts to the evolving nature of the encounter. Unlike static agreements that may be set in stone, dynamic negotiation recognizes that desires and boundaries can shift as the scene progresses. This adaptability is vital in breeding scenarios, where emotional and physical responses can change based on arousal levels, trust, and the unfolding dynamics between participants.

Key Principles of Dynamic Negotiation

- **Open Communication:** Encourage participants to express their desires, fears, and boundaries openly. This transparency fosters trust and ensures that everyone is on the same page.

- **Active Listening:** Pay attention to verbal and non-verbal cues. Participants should feel heard and validated, which enhances emotional safety.

- **Flexibility:** Be prepared to adjust plans based on the comfort levels and responses of all involved. Flexibility is essential for navigating unexpected situations or changes in mood.

+ **Mutual Respect:** Acknowledge and honor each participant's boundaries and preferences. This respect creates a safe environment conducive to exploration.

Negotiation Techniques for Breeding Scenes

1. Pre-Scene Negotiation Before engaging in a breeding scene, participants should have a thorough discussion about their desires, limits, and any potential health concerns. This discussion can include:

+ **Desire Mapping:** Each participant shares what they hope to experience during the scene. This can include specific fantasies, preferred activities, and emotional outcomes.

+ **Limit Setting:** Establish hard and soft limits. Hard limits are non-negotiable boundaries, while soft limits may be explored with caution. For example, a participant might have a hard limit against certain types of penetration but may be open to other forms of stimulation.

+ **Health and Safety:** Discuss any relevant health issues, including STIs, contraception, and emotional triggers. This dialogue ensures all participants feel safe and respected.

2. In-Scene Negotiation During the breeding scene, ongoing communication is vital. Participants should feel empowered to voice their comfort levels and desires as the scene unfolds. Techniques include:

+ **Check-Ins:** Regularly check in with each other. Simple questions like "How are you feeling?" or "Is this what you wanted?" can help gauge comfort levels and adjust the scene accordingly.

+ **Utilizing Safe Words:** Establish safe words that can be used to pause or stop the scene. This empowers participants to communicate discomfort without feeling pressured to justify their feelings.

+ **Observing Body Language:** Pay attention to non-verbal cues. A participant's body language can indicate pleasure or discomfort, providing insight into their emotional state.

COMMUNICATION AND NEGOTIATION

3. **Post-Scene Negotiation**   After the scene, participants should engage in a debriefing session to discuss their experiences. This reflection can enhance emotional intimacy and improve future encounters. Consider the following:

- **Emotional Check-In:** Discuss how each participant felt during the scene. This can include sharing highlights, challenges, and any unexpected feelings that arose.

- **Feedback Loop:** Provide constructive feedback to one another. Discuss what worked well and what could be improved for next time. This dialogue fosters growth and understanding.

- **Aftercare:** Engage in aftercare practices, such as cuddling, discussing the experience, or providing reassurance. Aftercare helps participants process their emotions and reinforces the bond created during the scene.

Addressing Common Negotiation Challenges

While dynamic negotiation is essential for successful breeding scenes, challenges can arise. Here are some common issues and strategies for addressing them:

- **Miscommunication:** Ensure clarity in discussions. Use direct language and avoid ambiguous terms. If misunderstandings occur, pause the scene to clarify intentions.

- **Unequal Power Dynamics:** Be aware of any power imbalances that may affect negotiation. Encourage all participants to voice their opinions and ensure that everyone feels empowered to express their desires and limits.

- **Emotional Triggers:** Participants may have past experiences that influence their current feelings. Encourage open dialogue about triggers and establish strategies for navigating these emotions during the scene.

Examples of Dynamic Negotiation in Action

To illustrate the principles of dynamic negotiation, consider the following scenarios:

Scenario 1: Pre-Scene Negotiation   Two partners discuss their desires for a breeding scene. One partner expresses a desire for multiple orgasms, while the other is interested in exploring roleplay. They agree to incorporate both elements but establish a safe word for the roleplay aspect, ensuring that either can pause the scene if it becomes uncomfortable.

Scenario 2: In-Scene Check-Ins During the scene, one partner feels overwhelmed and uses their safe word. The other partner immediately stops and checks in, asking what they can do to make the situation more comfortable. They discuss the feelings that arose and decide to shift focus to a different activity that feels more enjoyable.

Scenario 3: Post-Scene Reflection After a breeding scene, participants share their experiences. One partner expresses that they enjoyed the intensity but felt anxious about a specific moment. The other partner listens attentively and reassures them, discussing ways to enhance communication in future encounters.

Conclusion

Dynamic negotiation is a vital component of successful breeding scenes. By fostering open communication, practicing active listening, and remaining flexible, participants can create an environment that is safe, consensual, and deeply fulfilling. Embracing these techniques not only enhances the breeding experience but also strengthens the emotional connections between partners, paving the way for future adventures in the erotic lifestyle.

Creating the Perfect Breeding Environment

Setting the Scene

The Importance of Ambiance

Creating the right ambiance is a crucial aspect of establishing a breeding scene that heightens arousal and fosters intimacy. Ambiance encompasses the sensory elements of a space, including lighting, sound, scent, and temperature, which can profoundly affect the emotional and physical responses of those involved. This section will explore the significance of ambiance in breeding scenes, supported by theoretical insights and practical examples.

Theoretical Framework

Ambiance can be understood through various psychological theories, including the *Environmental Psychology Theory*, which posits that our surroundings influence our mood and behavior. The *Arousal Theory* suggests that certain environmental cues can stimulate physiological responses, enhancing sexual arousal. For instance, dim lighting may create a sense of intimacy and privacy, while soft music can evoke feelings of relaxation and pleasure.

$$A = f(E) \tag{7}$$

where A represents arousal and E symbolizes environmental factors. This equation illustrates that arousal is a function of the environment, emphasizing the need for a carefully curated ambiance in breeding scenes.

Key Elements of Ambiance

Lighting Lighting sets the mood for any intimate encounter. Soft, warm lighting can create a cozy and inviting atmosphere, while harsh fluorescent lights may evoke feelings of discomfort. Consider using dimmable lamps or candles to achieve the desired effect. For instance, a room illuminated by flickering candlelight can enhance the sensual experience, making the participants feel more connected and engaged.

Sound The auditory environment can significantly influence emotional states. Soft music, nature sounds, or even ambient noise can help create a relaxing backdrop. The choice of music should align with the participants' preferences and the desired mood. For example, a slow, sultry jazz playlist can evoke feelings of romance and desire, while rhythmic beats might energize the scene.

Scent Scent plays a powerful role in human attraction and memory. Incorporating essential oils, scented candles, or incense can enhance the ambiance and evoke specific emotions. For example, lavender is known for its calming properties, while ylang-ylang is often associated with sensuality. The use of pheromone-infused products can also stimulate attraction and arousal.

Temperature The physical comfort of the environment is essential for a pleasurable experience. An overly cold or hot space can distract participants and detract from the intimacy of the moment. Ideally, the temperature should be set to a comfortable level that allows for relaxation and engagement. Consider using blankets or soft fabrics to enhance comfort and warmth during the scene.

Practical Examples

To illustrate the importance of ambiance, consider the following scenarios:

- **Scenario One: A Romantic Night In**
  Imagine preparing a breeding scene at home. You dim the lights, light a few scented candles, and play soft music in the background. The room is warm and inviting, creating an atmosphere where both partners feel comfortable exploring their desires. This carefully crafted ambiance fosters a deeper connection and enhances the overall experience.

- **Scenario Two: An Outdoor Breeding Experience**
  For those who wish to take their breeding scene outside, consider the natural ambiance of a secluded area. The sounds of nature, the scent of fresh air, and

the warmth of the sun can create an exhilarating experience. However, it is crucial to ensure privacy and comfort, perhaps by bringing along blankets or cushions to sit on and setting boundaries regarding the space.

- **Scenario Three: A Public Play Party**
  In a public setting, the ambiance may be more challenging to control. However, selecting venues known for their sensual atmosphere—such as a dimly lit club with comfortable seating and soft music—can enhance the experience. Participants should communicate their needs and boundaries to navigate the shared space safely and enjoyably.

Conclusion

In conclusion, the importance of ambiance in breeding scenes cannot be overstated. By thoughtfully considering the elements of lighting, sound, scent, and temperature, participants can create an environment that enhances arousal, fosters intimacy, and ultimately leads to a more fulfilling experience. As you prepare for your breeding scenes, take the time to curate the ambiance, allowing it to reflect your desires and facilitate deeper connections with your partner(s). The right ambiance transforms a simple encounter into an unforgettable exploration of pleasure and intimacy.

Selecting the Right Location

Choosing the right location for breeding scenes is paramount to creating an atmosphere that enhances arousal, intimacy, and pleasure. The environment plays a significant role in setting the mood and can greatly influence the emotional and physical responses of all participants involved. This section delves into the various factors to consider when selecting a location, highlighting the importance of privacy, comfort, and the ability to engage fully in the experience.

1. Privacy and Discretion

One of the foremost considerations when selecting a location for breeding scenes is ensuring privacy. A private space allows participants to fully immerse themselves in the experience without fear of interruption or unwanted attention. This can be achieved through:

- **Home Environments:** Utilizing one's home can provide a familiar and comfortable setting. Consider transforming a bedroom or a designated playroom into a breeding sanctuary, complete with appropriate lighting, decor, and sensory elements.

- **Rented Spaces:** For those seeking a more neutral environment, consider renting a space specifically designed for adult activities. Many venues cater to erotic lifestyles, providing a safe and private atmosphere conducive to breeding scenes.

- **Outdoor Locations:** While outdoor breeding can be thrilling, it is essential to choose secluded areas where privacy is guaranteed, such as remote beaches, wooded areas, or private gardens. The thrill of being exposed can heighten arousal, but it must be balanced with the assurance of discretion.

2. Comfort and Accessibility

The physical comfort of all participants is crucial in fostering an enjoyable breeding experience. Factors to consider include:

- **Furniture and Layout:** Ensure that the location has comfortable seating or bedding that can accommodate various positions and activities. A spacious layout allows for movement and exploration, which can enhance the overall experience.

- **Temperature Control:** Maintaining a comfortable temperature is vital, as physical discomfort can detract from arousal. Consider locations with adjustable heating or cooling options.

- **Accessibility:** Ensure that the location is easily accessible for all participants, considering any mobility issues that may arise. Additionally, consider proximity to restrooms and other necessary amenities.

3. Sensory Elements

The ambiance of a location can significantly enhance the breeding experience. Engage the senses through:

- **Lighting:** Utilize soft, dim lighting to create a warm and inviting atmosphere. Consider using candles, fairy lights, or colored bulbs to set the mood. The right lighting can evoke feelings of intimacy and desire.

- **Sound:** Background music or ambient sounds can contribute to the overall experience. Choose music that resonates with the mood you wish to create—sensual, rhythmic beats or soft, melodic tunes can enhance arousal.

SETTING THE SCENE 45

- **Aromatherapy:** Incorporating scents through essential oils, incense, or scented candles can stimulate the senses and create a more immersive experience. Scents like vanilla, sandalwood, or jasmine are often associated with relaxation and arousal.

4. Safety Considerations

Safety must be a priority when selecting a location for breeding scenes. This encompasses both physical safety and emotional security:

- **Health and Hygiene:** Ensure that the location is clean and hygienic, particularly if multiple participants are involved. Have access to necessary supplies such as condoms, lubricants, and cleaning materials to maintain safety and comfort.

- **Emergency Preparedness:** Familiarize yourself with the location's emergency exits and procedures. Having a plan in place can alleviate anxiety and allow participants to focus on the experience.

- **Trust and Comfort:** All participants should feel safe and comfortable in the chosen location. If any individual feels uneasy about the space, it is essential to address these concerns before proceeding.

5. Examples of Ideal Locations

To illustrate the principles discussed, here are a few examples of ideal locations for breeding scenes:

- **Private Home:** A spacious bedroom with dim lighting, comfortable bedding, and personal touches that evoke intimacy can serve as an excellent breeding ground. Create a sensory haven with soft music and scented candles.

- **Hotel Suite:** Renting a hotel suite can provide an exciting escape. Look for suites with large beds, luxurious amenities, and the option for privacy. Ensure that the hotel has a discreet reputation to maintain confidentiality.

- **Outdoor Retreat:** A secluded cabin in the woods can offer the perfect blend of nature and privacy. Set up a comfortable area with blankets and pillows, and enjoy the sounds of nature as a backdrop to your breeding experience.

In conclusion, the selection of the right location for breeding scenes is crucial for maximizing pleasure and fostering deep connections. By prioritizing privacy, comfort, sensory engagement, and safety, participants can create an environment that enhances their breeding experiences, allowing them to fully explore their desires and fantasies.

Utilizing Props and Accessories

In the realm of breeding scenes, the thoughtful selection and use of props and accessories can significantly enhance the experience, creating an atmosphere that fosters deeper connections and heightened arousal. This section explores the various types of props and accessories that can be utilized, their psychological implications, and practical examples of how to incorporate them into your breeding scenes.

Types of Props and Accessories

Props and accessories can be categorized into several types, each serving unique purposes within the context of breeding scenes. These include:

- **Sensory Enhancers:** Items such as blindfolds, feathers, and ice cubes can heighten the sensory experience, intensifying pleasure and anticipation.

- **Fetish Gear:** Latex, leather, or other fetish wear can add an element of excitement and visual appeal, aligning with the aesthetic of breeding fantasies.

- **Sex Toys:** Vibrators, dildos, and other sex toys can augment physical stimulation, allowing for varied sensations and experiences.

- **Costumes and Roleplay Accessories:** Outfits that align with specific fantasies can enhance roleplay scenarios, deepening the immersion into the breeding scene.

- **Safety Tools:** Items such as condoms and dental dams are essential for maintaining sexual health and safety during breeding scenes.

Psychological Implications

The use of props and accessories in breeding scenes is not merely about physical pleasure; it also taps into the psychological aspects of arousal. The incorporation

SETTING THE SCENE 47

of props can trigger fantasies, enhance the feeling of submission or dominance, and create a more immersive experience. For instance, the act of wearing a blindfold can amplify sensations, as the removal of sight heightens other senses, making every touch feel more intense.

Furthermore, props can serve as symbols of trust and intimacy. When partners agree to use specific accessories, it signifies a level of comfort and understanding, fostering a deeper emotional connection. The act of selecting and preparing these items together can also serve as a bonding experience, enhancing the overall dynamic of the relationship.

Practical Examples

1. **Blindfolds and Sensory Deprivation:** The use of a blindfold can transform a breeding scene by removing visual stimuli, allowing partners to focus on touch, sound, and smell. Experimenting with different materials, such as silk or leather, can add to the experience. For example, a soft silk blindfold can evoke feelings of luxury and tenderness, while a leather blindfold may enhance the feeling of submission.

2. **Fetish Gear:** Incorporating fetish wear, such as corsets or harnesses, can amplify the visual aspect of a breeding scene. Wearing these items not only enhances the aesthetic but can also boost confidence and arousal. Consider using a strappy harness that emphasizes the body and creates a sense of vulnerability and desirability.

3. **Sex Toys:** The strategic use of sex toys can create layers of pleasure during breeding scenes. For example, a vibrating cock ring can provide additional stimulation for both partners, enhancing the experience of multiple loads. Alternatively, a prostate massager can be introduced for those exploring male anatomy, offering new dimensions of pleasure and orgasm control.

4. **Roleplay Accessories:** Costumes and roleplay accessories can facilitate the exploration of fantasies related to breeding. For instance, a nurse costume can introduce a playful dynamic, where one partner takes on a nurturing role, while the other submits to their care. This can create a context for breeding that feels safe and exciting.

5. **Safety Tools:** It is crucial to incorporate safety tools into breeding scenes. The use of condoms not only promotes sexual health but can also be integrated into the play itself. For instance, discussing the act of putting on a condom can serve as a form of foreplay, heightening anticipation before the breeding scene begins.

Conclusion

Incorporating props and accessories into breeding scenes can elevate the experience, transforming it into a multifaceted exploration of pleasure, intimacy, and fantasy. By understanding the types of props available, their psychological implications, and practical applications, partners can create a breeding environment that is not only safe but also deeply fulfilling. The key lies in open communication and mutual consent, ensuring that both partners feel comfortable and excited to explore the depths of their desires.

Utilizing props and accessories is an art that requires creativity and thoughtfulness, allowing for a rich tapestry of experiences that can enhance the overall breeding lifestyle. Embrace the possibilities, and let your imagination guide you in crafting unforgettable moments that resonate with your deepest desires.

Creating a Sensual and Arousal-Enhancing Atmosphere

Creating a sensual and arousal-enhancing atmosphere is essential for setting the stage for intimate experiences, particularly in breeding scenes. The environment in which these encounters take place can significantly influence emotional connection, arousal levels, and overall satisfaction. This section will explore various elements that contribute to an enticing atmosphere, focusing on lighting, scent, sound, and tactile sensations.

1. The Importance of Ambiance

Ambiance refers to the character and atmosphere of a space. In the context of breeding scenes, a well-crafted ambiance can heighten arousal and create a safe haven for exploration. The theory of environmental psychology suggests that our surroundings can profoundly impact our emotions and behaviors. Therefore, curating an inviting atmosphere can facilitate deeper connections and enhance the overall experience.

2. Selecting the Right Location

Choosing the right location is foundational in creating an intimate atmosphere. Whether it's a cozy bedroom, a secluded outdoor space, or a rented venue, the location should evoke feelings of safety and privacy. Consider the following factors when selecting a location:

- **Privacy:** Ensure the space is free from interruptions and prying eyes. This can be achieved through soundproofing, curtains, or a secluded outdoor area.

SETTING THE SCENE 49

- **Comfort:** The location should be physically comfortable, with appropriate furniture and temperature control. Soft bedding, plush pillows, and blankets can enhance comfort.

- **Accessibility:** Ensure that all participants can easily access the space without logistical issues. Consider any mobility needs and provide accommodations as necessary.

3. Utilizing Props and Accessories

Props and accessories can play a significant role in enhancing the sensual atmosphere. They can be visually stimulating, provide tactile pleasure, or serve specific functions during breeding scenes. Consider incorporating the following elements:

- **Textiles:** Use luxurious fabrics like silk, satin, or velvet for bedding and drapery to create a visually appealing and tactilely inviting environment.

- **Lighting:** Dim lighting or candles can create a warm, intimate glow. Consider using colored lights or lamps with adjustable brightness to set the mood.

- **Erotic Toys:** Introduce toys that align with the desires of all participants. This could include vibrators, dildos, or bondage gear, enhancing both visual and experiential elements of the scene.

4. Creating a Sensual and Arousal-Enhancing Atmosphere through Scent

Scent is a powerful sense that can evoke memories and emotions, making it a vital component of a sensual atmosphere. The use of aromatherapy can enhance arousal and create a welcoming environment. Consider the following:

- **Essential Oils:** Scents like jasmine, ylang-ylang, and sandalwood are known for their aphrodisiac properties. Diffusing these oils can create a romantic atmosphere.

- **Candles:** Scented candles not only provide soft lighting but also fill the space with enticing aromas. Choose candles made from natural wax and avoid synthetic fragrances to ensure a clean burn.

- **Personal Scents:** Encourage participants to wear scents that they find appealing. This personal touch can amplify attraction and create a unique sensory experience.

5. The Role of Sound in Sensual Atmosphere

Sound can profoundly influence mood and arousal. The right auditory backdrop can enhance intimacy and create a sense of connection. Consider the following elements:

- **Music:** Curate a playlist of sensual music that resonates with all participants. Genres like ambient, smooth jazz, or soft R&B can create an inviting atmosphere.

- **Nature Sounds:** Incorporating sounds of nature, such as ocean waves or birds chirping, can create a serene backdrop that promotes relaxation and intimacy.

- **Silence:** Sometimes, the absence of sound can be just as powerful. Embrace moments of silence to enhance the connection between participants, allowing for non-verbal communication and intimacy.

6. Incorporating Tactile Experiences

Tactile sensations can significantly enhance arousal and intimacy during breeding scenes. Consider the following techniques to engage the sense of touch:

- **Temperature Play:** Experiment with temperature by using warm oils for massage or cool objects to heighten sensitivity. This can create a dynamic and exciting sensory experience.

- **Textures:** Incorporate various textures through fabrics, toys, or even food. The contrast between soft, rough, smooth, and sticky can create a rich tactile experience.

- **Massage:** Begin the scene with sensual massages to enhance relaxation and intimacy. Focus on erogenous zones and explore different techniques to build arousal gradually.

7. Creating a Safe Space for Exploration

Ultimately, the atmosphere should foster a sense of safety and comfort. Establishing a safe space involves:

- **Clear Communication:** Encourage open dialogue about desires, boundaries, and consent. This transparency fosters trust and enhances the overall experience.

- **Aftercare:** Plan for aftercare to ensure emotional and physical well-being post-scene. This can include cuddling, gentle conversation, or sharing a meal.

- **Feedback:** After the experience, engage in a debriefing discussion to address what worked well and what could be improved. This practice reinforces trust and encourages future exploration.

In conclusion, creating a sensual and arousal-enhancing atmosphere is a multifaceted endeavor that requires attention to detail and consideration of all sensory experiences. By thoughtfully curating the environment, participants can fully immerse themselves in the breeding scene, fostering deeper connections and heightened pleasure. Embrace the art of ambiance, and let it transform your intimate encounters into unforgettable experiences.

Incorporating Sensory Experiences into Your Breeding Space

Creating an immersive breeding environment requires careful attention to the sensory experiences that will enhance arousal and connection between partners. The integration of various sensory elements can elevate the intensity of breeding scenes, allowing participants to delve deeper into their desires and fantasies. This section explores how to incorporate sensory experiences into your breeding space, focusing on sight, sound, touch, taste, and smell.

The Role of Sensory Stimulation

Sensory stimulation plays a crucial role in enhancing erotic experiences. According to research in psychology, engaging multiple senses can amplify emotional responses and increase the overall pleasure derived from intimate encounters. The theory of *multi-sensory integration* suggests that the brain processes information from different sensory modalities simultaneously, leading to a richer and more fulfilling experience.

$$P = f(S_1, S_2, S_3, S_4, S_5) \tag{8}$$

Where P represents pleasure, and S_1, S_2, S_3, S_4, S_5 correspond to sight, sound, touch, taste, and smell, respectively. The function f indicates that pleasure is a function of the combined sensory inputs, highlighting the importance of a well-rounded sensory experience.

Sight: Creating a Visually Stimulating Environment

Visual elements can significantly enhance the mood and ambiance of your breeding space. Consider the following techniques:

- **Lighting:** Use soft, dimmable lights or colored LED strips to create a warm and inviting atmosphere. The color red, for instance, is often associated with passion and desire.

- **Decor:** Incorporate sensual artwork, mirrors, and fabrics that evoke eroticism. Textured materials can add depth to the visual experience, enticing the eye and igniting the imagination.

- **Clothing:** Select outfits that accentuate the body and heighten arousal. Lingerie, costumes, or themed attire can visually stimulate both partners and set the tone for the scene.

Sound: Crafting an Auditory Experience

Sound can profoundly influence the atmosphere of your breeding space. Here are some suggestions for auditory stimulation:

- **Music:** Curate a playlist of sensual and erotic music that resonates with both partners. Consider genres like ambient, downtempo, or even classical pieces known for their romantic undertones.

- **Ambient Sounds:** Incorporate nature sounds, such as ocean waves or forest ambiance, to create a relaxing backdrop. This can help reduce anxiety and foster a deeper connection.

- **Voice:** Utilize soft whispers, moans, or even guided erotic narratives to enhance intimacy. The sound of your partner's voice can be incredibly arousing, deepening the emotional connection.

Touch: Enhancing Physical Connection

The sense of touch is paramount in breeding scenes, as it fosters intimacy and connection. Consider these elements:

- **Textures:** Introduce a variety of textures into your space, such as silk sheets, fur throws, or soft pillows. Experimenting with different materials can heighten tactile sensations during intimate moments.

SETTING THE SCENE

- **Temperature Play:** Incorporate warm oils, heated massage stones, or cool items like ice cubes to explore temperature variations. This can create contrasting sensations that amplify pleasure.

- **Massage:** Engage in sensual massages to enhance touch and relaxation. This not only builds anticipation but also fosters intimacy and trust between partners.

Taste: Exploring Flavorful Experiences

Taste can also play a vital role in enhancing sensory experiences during breeding scenes. Here are some ideas:

- **Edible Treats:** Incorporate fruits, chocolates, or whipped cream into your scenes. Feeding each other can create a playful and intimate dynamic, heightening arousal.

- **Flavored Lubricants:** Use flavored lubricants during oral activities to engage the sense of taste. This can add an exciting dimension to intimate encounters.

- **Beverages:** Consider serving aphrodisiac-infused drinks, such as wine or cocktails with exotic spices. The act of sharing a drink can enhance the overall experience.

Smell: Creating an Aromatic Atmosphere

The sense of smell is closely linked to memory and emotion, making it a powerful tool for enhancing breeding scenes. Here are some suggestions:

- **Aromatherapy:** Use essential oils or scented candles to create a calming and arousing environment. Scents like jasmine, ylang-ylang, and sandalwood are known for their aphrodisiac properties.

- **Personal Scents:** Embrace the natural scents of your bodies. Consider using pheromone-infused products to enhance attraction and intimacy.

- **Incense:** Burning incense can create a mystical atmosphere, enhancing the overall sensory experience. Choose scents that promote relaxation and arousal.

Combining Sensory Elements

To create a truly immersive breeding environment, consider combining sensory elements. For example, dim lighting paired with soft music and aromatic scents can create a tranquil atmosphere conducive to intimacy. Engaging multiple senses simultaneously can lead to heightened arousal and a deeper emotional connection.

Conclusion

Incorporating sensory experiences into your breeding space is essential for creating an environment that fosters intimacy and pleasure. By thoughtfully considering the elements of sight, sound, touch, taste, and smell, you can craft a breeding scene that resonates deeply with both partners. Experimenting with different combinations of sensory stimulation can lead to new heights of erotic exploration, ultimately enhancing your breeding lifestyle.

Techniques for Maximizing Pleasure

Foreplay and Teasing

Sensual Massage Techniques

Sensual massage is an intimate and powerful way to enhance the experience of breeding scenes, fostering deeper connections between partners while heightening arousal. This section will explore various techniques, theories, and practical applications of sensual massage that can be integrated into your breeding experiences.

Theoretical Foundations of Sensual Massage

Sensual massage is rooted in the understanding of human anatomy and the physiological responses to touch. The skin, being the largest organ, is rich with nerve endings that respond to various types of stimulation. According to [?], the sensation of touch activates the somatosensory cortex, which processes tactile information and can lead to feelings of pleasure and relaxation.

Moreover, the concept of *tactile communication* suggests that physical touch can convey emotions and intentions that words may fail to express [?]. By integrating sensual massage into breeding scenes, partners can communicate their desires and boundaries non-verbally, enhancing the overall experience.

Common Problems in Sensual Massage

While sensual massage can be an incredibly rewarding experience, several common issues may arise:

- **Discomfort or Pain:** If pressure is applied incorrectly, it can lead to discomfort. It is crucial to communicate openly about what feels good and what does not.

- **Lack of Connection:** If partners are not emotionally connected, the massage may feel mechanical rather than intimate. Building rapport and trust beforehand can mitigate this issue.

- **Distractions:** External factors such as noise or interruptions can break the mood. Creating a calming environment is essential for a successful sensual massage.

Techniques for Sensual Massage

To effectively incorporate sensual massage into your breeding scenes, consider the following techniques:

1. The Art of Touch The essence of sensual massage lies in the art of touch. Begin with light, feather-like strokes across the skin to awaken the senses. Gradually increase pressure as you gauge your partner's response. The *Swedish massage technique* is particularly effective, focusing on long, gliding strokes, kneading, and circular movements.

$$\text{Pressure} = \frac{\text{Force}}{\text{Area}} \quad (9)$$

Where pressure is the sensation felt by the receiver, force is the amount of pressure applied, and area is the surface area of contact. Adjusting the force and area can modify the sensation experienced, allowing for personalized pleasure.

2. Utilizing Oils and Lotions Incorporating massage oils or lotions can enhance the sensory experience by reducing friction and adding a fragrant element to the massage. Essential oils, such as lavender or ylang-ylang, can also promote relaxation and arousal. Always conduct a patch test to ensure there are no allergic reactions.

3. Focus on Erogenous Zones During sensual massage, pay special attention to erogenous zones, which are areas of the body that elicit heightened sexual arousal. These include:

- **Neck and Shoulders:** Gentle kneading can relieve tension and stimulate intimacy.

- **Inner Thighs:** Light strokes can build anticipation and heighten arousal.
- **Back:** Long strokes along the spine can create a sense of connection and relaxation.

4. Breathing Techniques Synchronizing breath with your partner can deepen the intimate experience. Encourage your partner to breathe deeply and slowly, matching your strokes to their inhalations and exhalations. This practice not only enhances relaxation but also fosters a sense of unity.

5. Experimenting with Temperature Using warm oils or incorporating hot stones can add an exciting element to sensual massage. Conversely, cold objects like ice cubes can stimulate the skin and create a thrilling contrast. Always ensure that temperature changes are safe and consensual.

Examples of Sensual Massage Routines

To illustrate the application of these techniques, consider the following routine:

1. **Set the Scene:** Dim the lights, play soft music, and ensure the environment is free from distractions.
2. **Start with Light Strokes:** Begin by gently caressing your partner's arms and legs, gradually building intimacy.
3. **Incorporate Oils:** Apply a warm oil to your hands and continue with long, flowing strokes on the back and shoulders.
4. **Focus on Erogenous Zones:** Transition to the neck and inner thighs, using varying pressure to enhance arousal.
5. **End with Deep Breathing:** Conclude the massage by guiding your partner to focus on their breath, creating a shared moment of intimacy.

Conclusion

Sensual massage is a powerful tool in the realm of breeding scenes, offering a pathway to deeper emotional connections and heightened pleasure. By understanding the theoretical foundations, addressing common issues, and employing effective techniques, you can create an unforgettable experience that enhances your breeding lifestyle. Remember that communication and consent are paramount, ensuring that both partners feel safe and cherished throughout the process.

Oral Stimulation Tips and Tricks

Oral stimulation is an art form that can elevate breeding scenes to new heights of pleasure and intimacy. When executed with intention and creativity, oral stimulation can enhance arousal, create deeper connections, and lead to multiple orgasms. This section will explore effective techniques, common challenges, and creative approaches to oral stimulation, ensuring that your experiences are both pleasurable and fulfilling.

Understanding the Anatomy

To master oral stimulation, it is essential to understand the anatomy involved. For individuals with a penis, key areas to focus on include:

- **Glans (Head):** The most sensitive part, rich in nerve endings.

- **Frenulum:** The band of tissue on the underside of the penis, highly sensitive and often a focal point for stimulation.

- **Shaft:** While less sensitive than the glans, the shaft can still provide pleasure through various techniques.

- **Scrotum:** The skin pouch that holds the testicles, sensitive to touch and temperature.

For individuals with a vulva, key areas include:

- **Clitoris:** The primary organ of sexual pleasure, containing numerous nerve endings.

- **Labia:** The outer and inner lips that can be stimulated through licking, sucking, or gentle nibbling.

- **G-Spot:** Located inside the vagina, often stimulated indirectly through the vaginal wall.

Techniques for Effective Oral Stimulation

1. **Varying Pressure and Speed** Experimenting with different levels of pressure and speed can lead to heightened sensations. Start with gentle strokes and gradually increase intensity. For example, when stimulating the glans, use a light touch with your tongue before applying more pressure as arousal builds.

2. **Incorporating Temperature Play** Temperature can significantly enhance the experience. Use ice cubes or warm drinks to create contrasting sensations. Alternating between warm and cool can heighten sensitivity and pleasure.

3. **Utilizing Your Hands** Incorporate your hands alongside oral stimulation. For example, while licking the shaft, use your hands to gently massage the testicles or the base of the penis. This combination can amplify pleasure and create a fuller experience.

4. **Exploring Different Techniques** Different techniques can lead to varied sensations. Here are a few to try:

- **The Lick and Suck:** Start with licking the glans and then transition to sucking gently. This combination stimulates both the surface and deeper areas.

- **The Circle:** Use your tongue to create circular motions around the sensitive areas, such as the frenulum or clitoris, to build anticipation.

- **The Squeeze:** While performing oral stimulation, use your lips to create a gentle squeezing motion, enhancing the sensation.

Common Challenges and Solutions

1. **Jaw Fatigue** One of the most common challenges during prolonged oral stimulation is jaw fatigue. To combat this, take breaks to massage your jaw or switch to a different position that allows for more comfortable movement.

2. **Saliva Management** Excess saliva can be a concern. Consider using flavored lubricants or gels to create a more enjoyable experience without the worry of messiness. Additionally, ensure proper hydration before engaging in oral play.

3. **Communication** Open communication is vital. Encourage your partner to express what feels good and what doesn't. Phrases like "That feels amazing" or "Can you try it this way?" can guide the experience, ensuring both partners are satisfied.

Incorporating Fantasy and Roleplay

Oral stimulation can be enhanced through fantasy and roleplay. Consider setting a scene that excites both partners. For instance, roleplaying as a seductive character can add a layer of eroticism to the experience. Use props or costumes to create an immersive environment that enhances arousal and pleasure.

Conclusion

Mastering oral stimulation is about exploration, creativity, and communication. By understanding anatomy, experimenting with techniques, and addressing common challenges, you can create unforgettable experiences that deepen connections and enhance pleasure. Remember, the journey of discovery is just as important as the destination, so embrace the process and enjoy every moment.

Incorporating Dirty Talk

Dirty talk is an essential component of many intimate encounters, especially in breeding scenes where the interplay of desire, power, and eroticism can be heightened through verbal expression. This section explores the nuances of dirty talk, its psychological underpinnings, and practical techniques to enhance your breeding experience.

The Psychology of Dirty Talk

Dirty talk serves multiple functions in sexual encounters. It can enhance arousal, deepen emotional connections, and facilitate communication about desires and boundaries. The psychological impact of dirty talk is rooted in its ability to:

- **Heighten Arousal:** Verbal expressions of desire can stimulate the imagination and increase physiological arousal. Research indicates that erotic language activates the brain's reward centers, releasing dopamine and enhancing pleasure (Sescousse et al., 2013).

- **Establish Power Dynamics:** In breeding scenarios, dirty talk can reinforce roles of dominance and submission. Phrases that assert control or express submission can deepen the psychological experience of the scene.

- **Foster Intimacy:** Sharing fantasies and desires verbally can create a sense of closeness and vulnerability, enhancing the emotional connection between partners.

Common Challenges with Dirty Talk

Despite its benefits, incorporating dirty talk can present challenges. Some common issues include:

- **Self-Consciousness:** Many individuals feel awkward or embarrassed when attempting to engage in dirty talk, fearing judgment or rejection.

- **Miscommunication:** Without clear communication, partners may misinterpret intentions, leading to discomfort or conflict.

- **Incompatibility:** Not everyone enjoys or feels comfortable with dirty talk. It is crucial to assess your partner's preferences and boundaries before incorporating it into your intimate life.

Techniques for Effective Dirty Talk

To successfully incorporate dirty talk into your breeding scenes, consider the following techniques:

- **Start Slow:** If you or your partner are new to dirty talk, begin with subtle compliments or suggestive phrases. Gradually increase the intensity as comfort levels grow. For example, you might start with, "You feel so good," before progressing to more explicit expressions of desire.

- **Use Sensory Language:** Engage your partner's senses by describing what you see, feel, and want. Phrases like, "I can't wait to feel you inside me," or "Your body drives me wild," can evoke vivid imagery and stimulate arousal.

- **Express Desires and Fantasies:** Share your fantasies openly. Phrases such as, "I want to feel you fill me up," or "Imagine us surrounded by others, completely lost in each other," can create a shared narrative that heightens excitement.

- **Incorporate Roleplay:** Roleplaying scenarios can be enhanced through dirty talk. If you are exploring a breeding scenario, you might say, "You're going to fill me with your seed, aren't you?" This not only reinforces the fantasy but also establishes the dynamic you wish to explore.

- **Use Affirmations:** Positive affirmations can enhance the experience. Statements like, "You make me feel so good," or "I love it when you take control," can boost confidence and deepen the connection between partners.

Examples of Dirty Talk in Breeding Scenes

Here are some practical examples of dirty talk tailored for breeding scenes:

- **Expressing Desire:** "I want you to fill me up completely. I crave every drop of you."

- **Encouraging Submission:** "You're going to let me take all of you, aren't you? You belong to me."

- **Building Anticipation:** "Just imagine how good it will feel when I'm full of you. I can't wait to experience it."

- **Reinforcing the Scene:** "You're going to make me a mother. I want you to give me everything you have."

Conclusion

Incorporating dirty talk into your breeding scenes can significantly enhance the erotic experience. By understanding its psychological impact, addressing common challenges, and employing effective techniques, you can create a more intimate and fulfilling connection with your partner. Remember to prioritize consent and communication, ensuring that both partners feel comfortable and excited to explore this aspect of their sexual expression. As you practice and experiment with dirty talk, you may find new depths of pleasure and connection within your breeding lifestyle.

Bibliography

[1] Sescousse, G., Redouté, J., & Dreher, J. C. (2013). The Functional Organization of the Reward Circuitry in the Human Brain. *Neuroscience and Biobehavioral Reviews*, 37(9), 1839-1850.

Utilizing Foreplay to Build Anticipation and Intensify Orgasms

Foreplay is an essential component of any erotic encounter, particularly in breeding scenes, where building anticipation can significantly enhance the overall experience. This section explores the various techniques and theories behind effective foreplay, emphasizing how it can be utilized to create a heightened sense of desire and lead to more intense orgasms.

The Psychological Impact of Foreplay

Foreplay serves not only as a physical warm-up but also as a psychological precursor to sexual activity. The anticipation generated during this phase can lead to increased arousal, making the eventual climax more satisfying. According to the *Dual Control Model* of sexual response, both excitatory and inhibitory processes play crucial roles in sexual arousal. Engaging in foreplay activates the excitatory processes, thereby enhancing the overall experience.

$$E = E_a - I_b \qquad (10)$$

Where:

- E = Overall arousal
- E_a = Excitatory factors (e.g., foreplay)
- I_b = Inhibitory factors (e.g., stress, anxiety)

Techniques for Building Anticipation

1. **Sensual Touch**: Begin with soft, lingering touches across the body. Focus on erogenous zones such as the neck, inner thighs, and lower back. The goal is to create a sense of connection and intimacy. Use varying pressures and speeds to keep your partner guessing and engaged.

2. **Teasing**: Engage in playful teasing by alternating between light touches and moments of withdrawal. For example, you might lightly brush your fingers against your partner's skin, only to pull away just as they begin to crave more. This technique can amplify desire and make the eventual contact more electrifying.

3. **Dirty Talk**: Verbal communication can be a powerful tool during foreplay. Whispering fantasies or desires into your partner's ear can stimulate their imagination and heighten arousal. Phrases that express longing or anticipation can create a thrilling atmosphere.

4. **Roleplay**: Incorporating elements of roleplay can enhance the foreplay experience. Assume different characters or scenarios that excite both partners, allowing for a deeper exploration of fantasies and desires.

5. **Gradual Undressing**: Instead of rushing into the physical act, take your time undressing each other. This act can be both intimate and erotic, allowing for prolonged eye contact and physical closeness. Each layer removed can symbolize a step deeper into intimacy.

Building Intensity through Foreplay

The key to intensifying orgasms lies in the careful orchestration of foreplay. Techniques such as edging can be particularly effective. Edging involves bringing your partner close to orgasm and then backing off, creating a cycle of heightened arousal. This method can be repeated multiple times, ultimately leading to a more explosive climax.

$$C = \sum_{n=1}^{N} A_n \qquad (11)$$

Where:

- C = Climax intensity
- A_n = Arousal level at each edging point
- N = Number of edging cycles

Each cycle of edging increases the overall arousal, leading to a more intense climax when finally allowed to release.

Common Problems and Solutions

While foreplay is generally a positive experience, some issues may arise:
  - **Disconnection**: If one partner feels disconnected or uninterested, it can dampen the mood. Address this by engaging in open communication about what feels good and what does not.
  - **Performance Anxiety**: Anxiety about performance can inhibit the enjoyment of foreplay. Encourage a relaxed atmosphere where both partners can express their needs without fear of judgment.
  - **Timing**: Some individuals may rush through foreplay, eager to reach the main event. Remind yourself and your partner that foreplay is an integral part of the experience and should not be hurried.

Conclusion

Utilizing foreplay effectively can significantly enhance the anticipation leading to breeding scenes, ultimately intensifying orgasms. By focusing on sensual touch, teasing, and communication, partners can create a dynamic and engaging experience that fosters deeper connections and satisfaction. Embrace the art of foreplay, and allow it to transform your intimate encounters into memorable and fulfilling experiences.

Exploring Roleplay and Fantasy in Breeding Scenes

Roleplay and fantasy serve as powerful tools in enhancing the depth and excitement of breeding scenes. They allow participants to step outside their everyday realities and explore desires that may otherwise remain unfulfilled. This section delves into the theoretical underpinnings of roleplay, the potential challenges it presents, and practical examples to inspire your breeding experiences.

Theoretical Framework of Roleplay

Roleplay can be understood through the lens of psychological theories such as *escapism* and *fantasy fulfillment*. Escapism refers to the tendency to seek distraction and relief from unpleasant realities, which can manifest in sexual contexts as individuals engage in roleplay to explore their fantasies. Fantasy fulfillment, as described by [?], suggests that engaging in fantasy can lead to increased sexual satisfaction and intimacy between partners.

The role of *narrative structure* in roleplay is also significant. According to [?], narratives provide a framework for understanding experiences and emotions, allowing participants to immerse themselves in their roles. In breeding scenes, narratives can range from the primal and instinctual to the more elaborate and structured, depending on the desires of those involved.

Challenges in Roleplay

While roleplay can enhance breeding scenes, it is not without its challenges. Miscommunication is a common issue, as participants may have different interpretations of roles or scenarios. Establishing clear boundaries and safe words is crucial to navigating these challenges. Additionally, emotional triggers may arise during roleplay, particularly if participants are exploring sensitive themes. It is essential to have a debriefing process in place to address any feelings that may surface.

Practical Examples of Roleplay Scenarios

To illustrate how roleplay can be integrated into breeding scenes, consider the following examples:

- **The Innocent Encounter:** One partner plays the role of a naive individual who is unaware of the breeding dynamics at play, while the other takes on a more experienced persona. This scenario can heighten the thrill of seduction and lead to a deeper exploration of power dynamics.

- **The Fertile Fantasy:** In this scenario, participants can roleplay as characters from a fantasy world where breeding is celebrated as a sacred act. This can involve elaborate costumes and settings, enhancing the immersive experience.

- **The Doctor-Patient Dynamic:** This roleplay involves one partner taking on the role of a medical professional who is conducting a fertility examination. This scenario can include elements of vulnerability and trust, as well as the excitement of exploring taboo themes.

- **The Group Breeding Party:** Participants can engage in a roleplay scenario where they are attending a breeding party, complete with multiple partners and a celebratory atmosphere. This allows for the exploration of group dynamics and the thrill of shared experiences.

Incorporating Roleplay into Breeding Scenes

To successfully incorporate roleplay into your breeding scenes, consider the following strategies:

1. **Communication is Key:** Before engaging in roleplay, have an open discussion about each partner's desires, boundaries, and any potential triggers. Establish safe words to ensure that everyone feels comfortable throughout the experience.

2. **Create a Detailed Narrative:** Develop a storyline that excites both partners. This could involve specific character traits, backgrounds, and motivations that enhance the roleplay experience. The more detailed the narrative, the more immersive the experience will be.

3. **Utilize Props and Costumes:** Incorporating props and costumes can significantly enhance the roleplay experience. Whether it's a simple outfit change or elaborate accessories, these elements can help participants fully embody their roles.

4. **Be Open to Exploration:** Roleplay is about exploration and experimentation. Be willing to adapt the scenario as it unfolds, allowing for spontaneous moments that can heighten arousal and connection.

5. **Debrief After the Scene:** After the roleplay experience, take time to discuss what worked, what didn't, and how each partner felt. This debriefing process can strengthen intimacy and trust, paving the way for future explorations.

Conclusion

Roleplay and fantasy play a vital role in enriching breeding scenes, offering a canvas for exploration and connection. By understanding the theoretical underpinnings, addressing potential challenges, and embracing creative scenarios, participants can elevate their experiences to new heights. As you embark on your breeding adventures, let your imagination guide you, and remember that the journey of discovery is just as important as the destination.

Mastering Multiple Loads

Understanding Male Anatomy

The Science Behind Multiple Orgasms

The phenomenon of multiple orgasms, particularly in the context of breeding scenes, is a captivating subject that intertwines physiological, psychological, and emotional dimensions of human sexuality. To understand this phenomenon, we must explore the underlying science, the factors that contribute to the ability to experience multiple orgasms, and the implications for enhancing pleasure in breeding scenarios.

Physiological Mechanisms

At the core of the ability to achieve multiple orgasms lies the anatomy of the human body, particularly the male reproductive system. The male orgasm is characterized by a series of physiological changes, including increased heart rate, muscle tension, and the release of various hormones. The primary hormone involved is oxytocin, often referred to as the "love hormone," which plays a significant role in bonding and emotional connection during sexual experiences.

The male orgasm can be divided into two phases: the emission phase and the expulsion phase. During the emission phase, sperm and seminal fluid are transported to the urethra, while the expulsion phase involves the rhythmic contractions of the pelvic muscles that propel semen out of the body. The ability to experience multiple orgasms is largely dependent on the refractory period—the time it takes for the body to recover after ejaculation.

$$R = \frac{T}{E} \qquad (12)$$

Where:

- R = Refractory period
- T = Time taken to recover
- E = Ejaculation

In some men, the refractory period can be as short as a few minutes, allowing for the possibility of achieving multiple orgasms in quick succession. Factors influencing the length of the refractory period include age, hormonal levels, and overall health.

The Role of Prostate Stimulation

Prostate stimulation can enhance the experience of multiple orgasms. The prostate, often referred to as the male G-spot, is a gland located just below the bladder and can be stimulated either externally or internally. When stimulated, the prostate can produce intense sensations and facilitate ejaculation without the typical refractory period associated with penile orgasm.

Research indicates that prostate stimulation can lead to a different type of orgasm, often described as a more profound and full-body experience. This type of orgasm may not be accompanied by the same ejaculatory response, allowing men to experience multiple orgasms more easily.

Psychological Factors

Psychological factors also play a crucial role in the experience of multiple orgasms. The mind's ability to focus on pleasure rather than performance can significantly enhance sexual experiences. Anxiety, stress, and performance pressure can inhibit sexual function and contribute to a longer refractory period.

Engaging in practices such as mindfulness, breath control, and visualization can help individuals to relax and enhance their sexual experiences. For example, focusing on the sensations in the body and practicing deep breathing can prolong arousal and facilitate the experience of multiple orgasms.

Techniques for Achieving Multiple Orgasms

There are various techniques that individuals can employ to increase the likelihood of experiencing multiple orgasms:

1. **Edging:** This technique involves bringing oneself close to orgasm and then stopping before ejaculation. This practice can help build arousal and intensity, making it easier to achieve multiple orgasms when the final release occurs.

2. **Kegel Exercises:** Strengthening the pelvic floor muscles through Kegel exercises can enhance control over ejaculation and increase the intensity of orgasms. Stronger pelvic muscles can lead to more powerful contractions during orgasm, facilitating multiple experiences.

3. **Prostate Play:** Incorporating prostate stimulation into sexual experiences can help men achieve orgasms that are distinct from penile ejaculation, allowing for multiple orgasms without the typical refractory period.

4. **Mindfulness and Relaxation Techniques:** Practicing mindfulness can help individuals remain present during sexual experiences, reducing anxiety and enhancing pleasure. Techniques such as deep breathing or guided imagery can facilitate a deeper connection to bodily sensations.

Conclusion

Understanding the science behind multiple orgasms reveals the intricate interplay of physiological, psychological, and emotional factors that contribute to this phenomenon. By exploring these dimensions, individuals can enhance their breeding experiences, fostering deeper connections and heightened pleasure. As we continue to unravel the complexities of human sexuality, embracing the potential for multiple orgasms can lead to more fulfilling and intimate encounters.

In summary, the journey toward mastering multiple orgasms is not solely a physical endeavor; it is an invitation to explore the depths of desire, connection, and pleasure. By integrating knowledge of anatomy, employing specific techniques, and nurturing a positive psychological environment, individuals can unlock the potential for extraordinary sexual experiences.

Training the Body for Enhanced Stamina

In the world of breeding scenes, stamina is not just a physical attribute; it is an essential component that enhances the overall experience for all participants. Training your body for enhanced stamina involves a combination of physical conditioning, mental preparation, and understanding your own sexual response. This section will delve into techniques, exercises, and practices that can help you build endurance, ensuring that you can fully engage in the pleasures of multiple loads.

Understanding Stamina

Stamina, in a sexual context, refers to the ability to sustain prolonged physical activity. It encompasses cardiovascular fitness, muscle endurance, and mental resilience. The relationship between physical fitness and sexual performance is well-documented, with studies indicating that individuals who engage in regular physical activity report higher levels of sexual satisfaction and endurance [?].

The Physiology of Stamina

To understand how to train for enhanced stamina, it is crucial to grasp the physiological mechanisms involved. The body relies on several systems during sexual activity:

- **Cardiovascular System:** A strong heart and efficient blood circulation are vital for maintaining energy levels and sustaining arousal. Increased heart rate during sexual activity enhances blood flow to the genitals, facilitating erections and arousal.

- **Muscular Endurance:** The pelvic floor muscles, including the pubococcygeus (PC) muscle, play a significant role in sexual function. Strengthening these muscles can lead to improved control over ejaculation and increased pleasure.

- **Mental Focus:** Stamina is not solely physical; mental endurance is equally important. The ability to maintain focus and manage arousal levels contributes to overall stamina.

Techniques for Building Stamina

1. **Cardiovascular Training** Engaging in regular cardiovascular exercise is essential for building stamina. Activities such as running, cycling, swimming, or dancing can improve heart health and increase lung capacity. Aim for at least 150 minutes of moderate-intensity aerobic exercise each week.

$$\text{VO}_2\text{max} = \frac{Q \cdot (A - V)}{W} \tag{13}$$

Where: - VO_2max is the maximum oxygen uptake, - Q is cardiac output, - A is arterial oxygen content, - V is venous oxygen content, - W is body weight.

Improving your VO_2 max through aerobic exercise will enhance your stamina, allowing you to engage in longer and more intense breeding sessions.

2. **Strength Training** Incorporating strength training into your routine can enhance muscular endurance. Focus on exercises that target the core and pelvic floor muscles, such as:

- **Kegel Exercises:** These exercises strengthen the pelvic floor muscles. To perform Kegels, identify your PC muscle (the muscle you use to stop urination). Contract this muscle for five seconds, then relax for five seconds. Repeat this cycle 10-15 times, three times a day.

- **Squats and Lunges:** These exercises build lower body strength, which is crucial for maintaining various positions during breeding scenes.

- **Planks:** Planks engage the core muscles, providing stability and endurance during prolonged activities.

3. **Interval Training** Incorporating interval training can enhance both cardiovascular and muscular endurance. This involves alternating between high-intensity bursts of activity and lower-intensity recovery periods. For example, during a workout, sprint for 30 seconds, followed by one minute of walking, and repeat this cycle for 20-30 minutes.

$$\text{Intensity} = \frac{\text{Duration of High-Intensity}}{\text{Total Duration}} \times 100\% \qquad (14)$$

Monitoring your intensity can help you gauge your progress and adjust your training accordingly.

4. **Mindfulness and Mental Training** Mental stamina is equally important in breeding scenes. Practicing mindfulness and meditation can enhance focus and reduce performance anxiety. Techniques such as deep breathing exercises can help you manage arousal levels and maintain control during intense experiences.

$$\text{Mindfulness Score} = \frac{\text{Focus Time}}{\text{Total Time}} \times 100\% \qquad (15)$$

Aim to increase your mindfulness score during intimate moments to enhance your overall stamina.

Common Challenges and Solutions

While training for enhanced stamina, you may encounter several challenges:

- **Fatigue:** It's essential to listen to your body. If you feel fatigued, allow for rest and recovery. Overtraining can lead to burnout, which may negatively impact your sexual performance.

- **Mental Barriers:** Performance anxiety can inhibit stamina. Engaging in open communication with your partner(s) can alleviate these fears and foster a supportive environment.

- **Injury:** Always prioritize safety. Use proper form during exercises and consider consulting a fitness professional to create a tailored training program.

Real-Life Examples

Consider the case of Alex and Jamie, a couple who wanted to enhance their breeding experiences. They implemented a training regimen that included:

- A combination of running and strength training three times a week.
- Daily Kegel exercises to strengthen their pelvic floor muscles.
- Mindfulness meditation sessions to improve mental focus and reduce anxiety.

After several weeks, they reported significant improvements in their stamina and overall sexual satisfaction. Their ability to engage in extended breeding scenes deepened their connection and heightened their pleasure.

Conclusion

Training the body for enhanced stamina is a multifaceted approach that involves physical conditioning, mental preparation, and a commitment to continuous improvement. By incorporating cardiovascular training, strength exercises, interval training, and mindfulness practices into your routine, you can build the stamina needed to fully enjoy the pleasures of breeding scenes. Remember, the journey to enhanced stamina is personal; take the time to explore what works best for you and your partner(s), ensuring that every encounter is fulfilling and pleasurable.

Exploring Prostate Stimulation

Prostate stimulation, often referred to as the "male G-spot," can enhance sexual pleasure and intensify orgasms. This section delves into the anatomy of the prostate, the techniques for effective stimulation, and the potential benefits and challenges associated with this practice.

Anatomy of the Prostate

The prostate is a walnut-sized gland located approximately 2-3 inches inside the rectum, on the anterior wall. It plays a crucial role in the male reproductive system by producing seminal fluid, which nourishes and transports sperm. The prostate is rich in nerve endings, making it highly sensitive to touch.

$$\text{Prostate Location} \approx \text{Rectal Depth} - 2.5 \text{ inches} \qquad (16)$$

Understanding its position is essential for effective stimulation. The prostate can be accessed through the rectum, and gentle pressure can create pleasurable sensations.

Techniques for Prostate Stimulation

Several techniques can be employed to stimulate the prostate effectively. Here are some of the most common methods:

- **Fingers:** Using well-lubricated fingers, insert one or two fingers into the rectum, curving them gently towards the front of the body. Apply pressure on the prostate, using a "come here" motion to stimulate the gland.

- **Prostate Massagers:** Specialized toys designed for prostate stimulation can provide targeted pressure. These devices often have a curve that allows for easy access to the prostate. Look for massagers with varying speeds and vibrations to enhance pleasure.

- **Vibrators:** Incorporating a vibrating device can amplify sensations. Experiment with different settings to discover what feels best for you or your partner.

- **Anal Play:** Combining anal penetration with prostate stimulation can heighten arousal. The pressure from anal penetration can create a fuller sensation while stimulating the prostate.

Benefits of Prostate Stimulation

The benefits of prostate stimulation extend beyond mere pleasure. Engaging in this practice can lead to:

- **Intensified Orgasms:** Many individuals report that prostate orgasms are more intense than penile orgasms, often resulting in a deeper and more fulfilling release.

- **Enhanced Sexual Pleasure:** Regular prostate stimulation can increase overall sexual enjoyment, adding variety to sexual experiences.

- **Improved Ejaculatory Control:** Learning to control the sensations associated with prostate stimulation can lead to better ejaculatory control and longer-lasting sexual encounters.

- **Health Benefits:** Some studies suggest that regular prostate stimulation may reduce the risk of prostate-related health issues, including prostatitis and benign prostatic hyperplasia (BPH).

Challenges and Considerations

While prostate stimulation can be pleasurable, it is essential to approach it with care. Some challenges may include:

- **Discomfort or Pain:** Not everyone will find prostate stimulation pleasurable. It is crucial to listen to your body and communicate with your partner. If discomfort occurs, stop and reassess.

- **Hygiene:** Ensuring cleanliness is vital for anal play. Use gloves or condoms on toys to maintain hygiene and reduce the risk of infections.

- **Mental Barriers:** Some individuals may have mental blocks regarding anal play or prostate stimulation. Open communication and gradual exploration can help overcome these barriers.

Practical Examples

To illustrate the effectiveness of prostate stimulation, consider the following scenarios:

- **Solo Exploration:** A person may begin by using a finger or a prostate massager while relaxing in a bath. The warm water can help ease tension, making the experience more enjoyable. Starting slowly and gradually increasing pressure can lead to heightened arousal.

- **Partnered Play:** During intimate moments, one partner may focus on stimulating the prostate while the other enjoys oral sex or clitoral stimulation. This combination can create a multi-layered experience that enhances pleasure for both partners.

- **Using Toys:** A couple might incorporate a vibrating prostate massager into their routine. One partner can control the settings while the other focuses on relaxation and pleasure, allowing for a shared experience that builds intimacy.

In conclusion, exploring prostate stimulation can significantly enhance sexual experiences. By understanding the anatomy, employing effective techniques, and addressing potential challenges, individuals can unlock new levels of pleasure and intimacy. Whether engaging in solo exploration or partnered play, the journey into prostate stimulation can be both fulfilling and rewarding.

Techniques for Controlling Ejaculation and Delaying Orgasm

Controlling ejaculation and delaying orgasm are essential techniques for enhancing pleasure in breeding scenes. These skills not only prolong the sexual experience but also deepen intimacy and connection between partners. This section explores various techniques and theories that can aid in mastering these abilities.

Understanding Ejaculation Control

Ejaculation is a complex physiological process influenced by both psychological and physical factors. The ability to control ejaculation involves understanding the body's responses and recognizing the stages leading to orgasm. The male sexual response cycle typically includes the following phases:

1. **Arousal:** Increased blood flow to the genitals, heightened sensitivity.

2. **Plateau:** Intensified arousal, increased heart rate, and muscle tension.

3. **Orgasm:** The peak of sexual pleasure, leading to ejaculation.

4. **Resolution:** The body gradually returns to its unaroused state.

By focusing on the plateau phase, individuals can learn to delay orgasm through various techniques.

Techniques for Delaying Orgasm

1. **The Start-Stop Technique** The start-stop technique involves alternating between periods of stimulation and pauses. This method allows the individual to become aware of their arousal levels and manage them effectively.

- **Implementation:** During sexual activity, when nearing the point of ejaculation, stop all stimulation. Breathe deeply and allow the arousal to subside slightly before resuming.

- **Benefits:** This technique can enhance control over ejaculation and increase overall pleasure.

2. **The Squeeze Technique** The squeeze technique involves applying pressure to the penis at the base or the head when ejaculation feels imminent.

- **Implementation:** When approaching orgasm, the partner can gently squeeze the shaft or the glans, temporarily halting the urge to ejaculate.

- **Benefits:** This method can significantly prolong sexual activity and intensify subsequent orgasms.

3. **Kegel Exercises** Kegel exercises strengthen the pelvic floor muscles, which can enhance control over ejaculation.

- **Implementation:** To perform Kegel exercises, identify the pelvic floor muscles by stopping urination midstream. Once identified, contract these muscles for 5 seconds, then relax for 5 seconds. Aim for three sets of 10 repetitions daily.

- **Benefits:** Strengthening these muscles can lead to improved control during sexual activities and more powerful orgasms.

4. **Edging** Edging is the practice of bringing oneself or a partner close to orgasm and then backing off before climaxing.

- **Implementation:** Engage in sexual activity until nearing orgasm, then either stop or switch to a less stimulating activity. Repeat this process several times before allowing ejaculation.

- **Benefits:** This technique builds sexual tension, leading to more intense orgasms when finally released.

Theoretical Considerations

The ability to control ejaculation is not merely a physical skill but also a psychological one. Anxiety and performance pressure can significantly impact sexual performance. Understanding the following theories can aid in developing these skills:

1. **Cognitive Behavioral Techniques** Cognitive-behavioral techniques focus on changing negative thought patterns associated with sexual performance. By reframing thoughts and reducing anxiety, individuals can enhance their sexual experience.

2. **Mindfulness and Sensate Focus** Mindfulness practices encourage individuals to focus on the present moment, enhancing awareness of bodily sensations. Sensate focus exercises involve partners taking turns to explore each other's bodies without the goal of orgasm, fostering deeper connection and relaxation.

Common Challenges

Mastering ejaculation control can come with challenges, including anxiety, overthinking, and performance pressure. Here are some common issues and potential solutions:

- **Anxiety:** Performance anxiety can hinder the ability to control ejaculation. Practicing relaxation techniques, such as deep breathing or meditation, can mitigate this issue.

- **Overstimulation:** In some cases, heightened sensitivity may lead to premature ejaculation. Employing the start-stop technique or Kegel exercises can help regain control.

- **Communication:** Open communication with partners about desires and boundaries can alleviate pressure and enhance the overall experience.

Conclusion

Controlling ejaculation and delaying orgasm are vital skills that can significantly enhance the breeding experience. By employing techniques such as the start-stop method, squeeze technique, Kegel exercises, and edging, individuals can cultivate greater intimacy and pleasure. Understanding the psychological aspects of sexual performance and addressing common challenges will further support the journey towards mastering these techniques. Embrace the process, and enjoy the exploration of your desires.

The Art of Edging and Building Intensity in Breeding Scenes

Edging, often referred to as orgasm denial or control, is a powerful technique that can significantly enhance the intensity and pleasure of breeding scenes. This practice involves bringing oneself or a partner to the brink of orgasm and then stopping or reducing stimulation before climaxing. The psychological and physiological effects of edging can lead to heightened arousal, more intense orgasms, and a deeper connection between partners.

Understanding Edging

At its core, edging is about mastering the balance between pleasure and restraint. The act of bringing oneself close to the edge of orgasm activates various physiological responses, including increased heart rate, heightened sensitivity, and intensified emotional connection. The anticipation built during edging can create a more profound experience when the eventual release occurs.

Theoretical Framework

The theory behind edging can be linked to the concept of **sexual tension**. Sexual tension is a state of heightened arousal that occurs when individuals are in a prolonged state of anticipation. According to the *Sexual Response Cycle* proposed by Masters and Johnson, the phases of excitement, plateau, orgasm, and resolution can be manipulated through edging. By extending the plateau phase, partners can experience a more intense climax when they finally allow themselves to release.

$$\text{Intensity of Orgasm} \propto \text{Duration of Plateau Phase} \quad (17)$$

This equation suggests that the longer the plateau phase is maintained, the more intense the subsequent orgasm will be. Thus, incorporating edging into breeding scenes can enhance the overall experience.

Practical Techniques for Edging

1. **Communication and Consent**: Before engaging in edging, it is crucial to have open discussions with your partner(s) about desires, limits, and safe words. Establishing clear communication ensures that everyone involved is comfortable and consenting to the experience.
2. **Gradual Stimulation**: Start with gentle stimulation, whether through manual, oral, or penetrative methods. Pay attention to your partner's responses, adjusting the pace and intensity based on their feedback.
3. **Recognizing the Edge**: Partners should learn to recognize the physical signs that indicate they are nearing orgasm. These can include changes in breathing patterns, muscle tension, and vocalizations.
4. **Controlled Release**: Once the edge is reached, reduce stimulation to prevent climax. This can be achieved by slowing down movements, changing positions, or focusing on different erogenous zones.
5. **Building Anticipation**: Use verbal cues or dirty talk to enhance the psychological aspect of edging. Phrases that emphasize the desire to climax or the pleasure of waiting can amplify arousal.

Examples of Edging in Breeding Scenes

- **Solo Edging**: A person can explore their body through self-stimulation, using toys designed for prolonged pleasure. Techniques such as alternating between vigorous and gentle stimulation can help maintain the edge.
- **Partnered Edging**: In a breeding scene, one partner may take the lead, controlling the pace and intensity of stimulation. For instance, during penetrative sex, one partner may withdraw just before climax, allowing the other to experience the build-up of pleasure without release.
- **Roleplay Dynamics**: Incorporating roleplay can enhance the experience of edging. For example, in a dominant/submissive dynamic, the dominant partner may dictate when the submissive partner can or cannot climax, adding an element of power exchange that intensifies the experience.

Common Challenges and Solutions

While edging can be a thrilling addition to breeding scenes, it may come with challenges. Here are some common issues and how to address them:

- **Frustration**: Partners may feel frustrated if they are repeatedly brought to the edge without release. To mitigate this, establish a safe word or signal that allows either partner to request a release if the experience becomes overwhelming.

- **Loss of Arousal**: Sometimes, prolonged edging can lead to a decrease in arousal. To counteract this, incorporate varied stimulation techniques, such as changing the rhythm or introducing new sensations to keep the experience engaging.

- **Communication Breakdowns**: Misunderstandings about boundaries or desires can occur. Regular check-ins during the scene can help ensure that both partners feel safe and satisfied.

Conclusion

The art of edging is a valuable technique for building intensity in breeding scenes. By understanding the physiological and psychological aspects of edging, partners can enhance their experiences, leading to more profound connections and heightened pleasure. Remember that the key to successful edging lies in communication, consent, and a willingness to explore the boundaries of pleasure together. Embrace the journey of anticipation, and allow the eventual release to become a celebration of your shared desires.

Strategies for Managing Multiple Participants

Solo Breeding

Techniques for Self-Stimulation

Self-stimulation, often referred to as masturbation, is a fundamental aspect of sexual exploration and pleasure. This section delves into various techniques that can enhance the experience, particularly in the context of breeding scenes. Understanding the mechanics of self-stimulation not only increases personal pleasure but also fosters a deeper connection with one's own body, paving the way for more fulfilling experiences with partners.

Understanding the Physiology of Self-Stimulation

Before diving into specific techniques, it's essential to understand the physiological responses involved in self-stimulation. The process typically involves the following stages:

- **Arousal:** This is the initial phase where physical and psychological stimuli lead to increased blood flow to the genitals, resulting in erection in males and lubrication in females.

- **Plateau:** During this phase, sexual tension builds, and the body prepares for orgasm. The heart rate increases, and breathing becomes more rapid.

- **Orgasm:** This is the peak of sexual pleasure, characterized by rhythmic contractions of the pelvic muscles and ejaculation in males, or intense contractions of the vaginal muscles in females.

- **Resolution:** Following orgasm, the body gradually returns to its normal state, often accompanied by feelings of relaxation and satisfaction.

Understanding these stages can help individuals tailor their self-stimulation techniques to maximize pleasure.

Techniques for Enhanced Self-Stimulation

1. Varying Grip and Pressure   One of the simplest yet most effective techniques involves varying the grip and pressure applied during self-stimulation. For example:

- **Light Touch:** Start with a gentle caress of the genitals, focusing on sensitive areas such as the glans or clitoris. This can heighten sensitivity and build anticipation.

- **Firm Grip:** Gradually increase the pressure, using a firmer grip to stimulate the shaft or the base of the penis. This can create a contrasting sensation that enhances pleasure.

- **Alternating Techniques:** Switch between light and firm touches to keep the experience dynamic and exciting.

2. Utilizing Lubrication   Lubrication is crucial for enhancing sensations during self-stimulation. Different types of lubricants can provide varied experiences:

- **Water-Based Lubricants:** These are versatile and safe to use with condoms and sex toys. They provide a smooth glide but may require reapplication.

- **Silicone-Based Lubricants:** These last longer and provide a slick sensation, making them ideal for extended sessions.

- **Natural Oils:** Coconut oil or almond oil can offer a luxurious feel, but it's essential to note that they are not safe to use with latex condoms.

Experimenting with different lubricants can enhance the tactile experience and lead to more intense orgasms.

3. **Incorporating Toys** Sexual toys can elevate self-stimulation to new heights. Here are some examples:

- **Vibrators:** These can be used on various erogenous zones, including the clitoris, nipples, or perineum. The vibrations can stimulate nerve endings, enhancing arousal and pleasure.

- **Masturbation Sleeves:** These devices can mimic the sensations of penetrative sex, providing a unique experience that can be particularly satisfying during solo breeding scenarios.

- **Anal Toys:** For those interested in exploring anal stimulation, anal beads or prostate massagers can add a thrilling dimension to self-stimulation.

4. **Exploring Fantasy and Roleplay** Engaging the mind is just as important as physical stimulation. Incorporating fantasy and roleplay into self-stimulation can enhance arousal significantly:

- **Visual Aids:** Watching erotic films or reading erotic literature can stimulate the imagination and heighten arousal.

- **Roleplay Scenarios:** Creating scenarios that involve breeding dynamics can add excitement. For instance, imagining oneself in a breeding club or a scenario involving multiple partners can amplify the experience.

5. **Breathing Techniques** Breathing plays a crucial role in enhancing sexual pleasure. Practicing controlled breathing can help individuals maintain arousal and prolong the experience:

- **Deep Breathing:** Taking slow, deep breaths can help relax the body and heighten awareness of sensations.

- **Paced Breathing:** Synchronizing breath with movements can create a rhythm that enhances pleasure. For instance, inhale while applying pressure and exhale during release.

Addressing Common Challenges

While self-stimulation can be pleasurable, individuals may encounter challenges such as difficulty reaching orgasm or feelings of guilt. Here are some strategies to address these issues:

1. **Difficulty Reaching Orgasm**   If reaching orgasm proves challenging, consider the following:

- **Relaxation Techniques:** Stress and anxiety can impede sexual pleasure. Engaging in relaxation techniques such as meditation or yoga can help ease tension.

- **Experimenting with Techniques:** If certain techniques aren't effective, don't hesitate to try new methods or combinations to discover what works best for you.

2. **Guilt or Shame**   Feelings of guilt or shame regarding self-stimulation can stem from societal norms or personal beliefs. To overcome these feelings:

- **Education:** Understanding that self-stimulation is a normal and healthy part of human sexuality can help alleviate guilt.

- **Affirmations:** Practicing positive affirmations about one's sexuality can foster a more accepting attitude toward self-exploration.

Conclusion

Self-stimulation is a vital aspect of sexual health and exploration. By employing various techniques, individuals can enhance their experiences, paving the way for deeper connections with themselves and their partners. Embracing self-exploration not only enriches personal pleasure but also prepares individuals for more fulfilling breeding scenes in the future. Remember, the journey of self-discovery is as important as the destination, and each experience contributes to a more profound understanding of one's desires and pleasures.

Solo Breeding Accessories and Toys

In the realm of solo breeding, the right accessories and toys can significantly enhance the experience, allowing for exploration, pleasure, and self-discovery. This section delves into the various tools available for solo practitioners, their benefits, and how they can be integrated into your breeding scenes.

SOLO BREEDING

Types of Solo Breeding Accessories

1. Masturbation Devices Masturbation devices are essential for enhancing solo breeding experiences. These can range from simple strokers to more complex automated devices. The key to selecting the right device lies in understanding personal preferences and desired sensations.

- **Strokers:** These handheld devices mimic the sensations of penetrative sex. They come in various textures and materials, allowing users to select one that aligns with their fantasy.

- **Fleshlights:** A popular choice, Fleshlights offer realistic sensations and are designed to resemble anatomical features. They can be used with lubricants to enhance pleasure.

- **Automated Masturbators:** These devices provide hands-free stimulation and often come with adjustable settings for speed and intensity, allowing for a tailored experience.

2. Vibrators Vibrators can be an exciting addition to solo breeding scenes, providing additional stimulation that enhances arousal. They can be used on various erogenous zones, including the penis, perineum, and even the prostate.

- **Penis Vibrators:** Designed specifically for the penis, these vibrators can provide targeted stimulation and can be used in conjunction with other devices for heightened pleasure.

- **Prostate Massagers:** These toys are designed to stimulate the prostate, often resulting in intense orgasms. They can be used alone or alongside other devices for a more comprehensive experience.

3. Lubricants While not a toy in the traditional sense, lubricants are crucial for enhancing pleasure during solo breeding. They reduce friction and can intensify sensations, making the experience more enjoyable.

- **Water-Based Lubricants:** These are versatile and safe to use with most toys. They are easy to clean and provide a natural feel.

- **Silicone-Based Lubricants:** Offering a longer-lasting glide, silicone-based lubricants are great for use in the bath or shower but should not be used with silicone toys.

- **Hybrid Lubricants:** Combining elements of both water and silicone, hybrid lubricants offer the best of both worlds, providing a smooth, long-lasting experience.

Incorporating Accessories into Solo Breeding

The integration of these accessories into solo breeding can take various forms, depending on individual preferences and the desired outcomes. Here are some techniques to maximize pleasure:

1. Layering Sensations Using multiple toys simultaneously can create a more immersive experience. For instance, using a stroker while applying a prostate massager can provide dual stimulation, enhancing the overall intensity of the session.

2. Experimenting with Settings For automated devices, experimenting with different speed and intensity settings can help discover personal preferences. Adjusting the settings throughout the session can also prolong arousal and lead to more powerful orgasms.

3. Incorporating Fantasy Utilizing toys that align with specific fantasies can elevate the experience. For example, a user might select a toy that mimics a particular partner or scenario, allowing for a more fulfilling solo breeding session.

Safety and Hygiene Considerations

When engaging in solo breeding with accessories, safety and hygiene are paramount. Here are essential guidelines to follow:

- **Cleaning Toys:** Always clean toys before and after use with appropriate cleaners. This helps prevent infections and maintains the longevity of the device.

- **Using Condoms:** For shared toys or to enhance cleanliness, consider using condoms on toys. This not only simplifies cleanup but also adds an extra layer of safety.

- **Checking for Damage:** Regularly inspect toys for wear and tear. Damaged toys can cause injury or discomfort, so replace them as necessary.

Conclusion

In summary, the right accessories and toys can significantly enhance the solo breeding experience. By selecting appropriate devices, incorporating them effectively, and adhering to safety guidelines, individuals can explore their desires and achieve satisfying outcomes. Whether through the use of strokers, vibrators, or lubricants, the journey of solo breeding can be both pleasurable and fulfilling, allowing for deeper connections with oneself and one's desires.

Solo Breeding Safety and Hygiene

When engaging in solo breeding scenes, prioritizing safety and hygiene is essential to ensure a pleasurable and healthy experience. This section will explore the critical aspects of safety and hygiene, providing practical advice and considerations for individuals who wish to embark on solo breeding adventures.

Understanding the Importance of Hygiene

Maintaining proper hygiene during solo breeding is crucial for several reasons:

- **Health Risks:** Engaging in sexual activities without adequate hygiene can lead to infections, such as urinary tract infections (UTIs) or sexually transmitted infections (STIs). Proper cleaning before and after activities minimizes these risks.

- **Enhanced Pleasure:** A clean environment and body can enhance the overall experience, allowing for greater relaxation and enjoyment.

- **Psychological Comfort:** Knowing that you are practicing good hygiene can improve mental well-being, allowing you to fully immerse yourself in the experience without distractions or concerns.

Pre-Scene Preparations

Before diving into your solo breeding session, consider the following preparatory steps:

1. **Personal Hygiene:**
    - Showering or bathing before your session is essential. Clean all areas of your body, particularly the genitals, to remove any bacteria or sweat that may cause discomfort or infection.

- Consider using gentle, unscented soaps to avoid irritation, especially for sensitive skin.

2. **Environment Cleanliness:**

    - Ensure that your chosen space is clean and free from dust or allergens. Wipe down surfaces with disinfectant wipes to eliminate any potential contaminants.
    - Create a comfortable and inviting atmosphere by decluttering the area and adding elements such as soft lighting, comfortable bedding, or scented candles (ensuring they are safe for use).

3. **Preparation of Accessories:**

    - If you plan to use toys or accessories, clean them thoroughly according to the manufacturer's instructions. Use warm water and mild soap or a designated toy cleaner.
    - Ensure that any items you plan to use are in good condition, free from cracks or damage that could lead to injury or infection.

During the Scene: Safe Practices

While engaged in solo breeding, maintaining safety and hygiene is paramount:

- **Use of Lubrication:**

    - Always use a suitable lubricant to reduce friction and enhance pleasure. Opt for water-based lubricants for easy cleanup and to prevent irritation.
    - Avoid using oils or lotions not designed for sexual activity, as they can cause irritation or damage to latex condoms or toys.

- **Monitoring Physical Responses:**

    - Pay attention to your body's signals. If you experience discomfort or pain, stop immediately and assess the situation.
    - Be aware of any changes in your body, such as unusual irritation or soreness, and address them promptly.

- **Condom Use:**

- Consider using condoms on toys or during self-penetration to maintain hygiene and ease of cleanup. Condoms can also help prevent the spread of bacteria.
- If you are using multiple toys or switching between different types of stimulation, change condoms between uses to avoid cross-contamination.

Post-Scene Hygiene and Care

After completing your solo breeding scene, follow these steps to maintain hygiene and safety:

1. **Clean Yourself:**

    + Shower again after your session to wash away any bodily fluids and bacteria. Pay special attention to the genital area.
    + If showering immediately is not possible, use unscented wipes to clean yourself until you can wash properly.

2. **Clean Your Toys:**

    + Clean all toys and accessories immediately after use. Follow the same cleaning procedures as before, ensuring they are thoroughly disinfected.
    + Store your toys in a clean, dry place, preferably in a dedicated bag or container to keep them free from dust and contaminants.

3. **Reflect on the Experience:**

    + Take a moment to reflect on your session. Consider what you enjoyed, what you might want to change next time, and any feelings that arose during the experience.
    + Journaling about your experience can help you process your emotions and enhance future solo breeding adventures.

Addressing Common Concerns

+ **Infection Concerns:**

    - If you notice any signs of infection, such as unusual discharge, itching, or discomfort, seek medical advice promptly. Early intervention can prevent further complications.

- **Mental Well-being:**
  - Engaging in solo breeding can evoke a range of emotions. If you experience feelings of guilt or anxiety, consider discussing these feelings with a trusted friend or a professional therapist specializing in sexual health.
- **Self-Exploration:**
  - Solo breeding is an opportunity for self-exploration and understanding your desires. Embrace this time as a chance to learn more about your body and what brings you pleasure.

In conclusion, maintaining safety and hygiene during solo breeding is essential for a pleasurable and healthy experience. By following these guidelines, individuals can create a safe and enjoyable environment that fosters exploration and satisfaction. Remember, the key to a fulfilling solo breeding experience lies in preparation, mindfulness, and self-care.

Developing Different Roles and Characters for Solo Breeding

In the realm of solo breeding, the exploration of different roles and characters can significantly enhance the experience, allowing individuals to delve deeper into their fantasies and desires. This section will explore the psychological underpinnings of role-playing, the benefits of character development, and practical examples to inspire your solo breeding sessions.

The Psychology of Role-Playing

Role-playing taps into the fundamental human desire for exploration and creativity. According to [?], engaging in role-play allows individuals to step outside their everyday identities, exploring aspects of themselves that may remain dormant in conventional scenarios. This can lead to heightened arousal, increased pleasure, and a deeper emotional connection to the experience.

Benefits of Character Development

Creating distinct characters for solo breeding can provide numerous benefits:

- **Enhanced Fantasy Engagement:** By embodying different personas, you can immerse yourself more fully in your fantasies, making the experience more vivid and exciting.

- **Exploration of Desires:** Role-playing allows you to explore desires that may not align with your everyday self, offering a safe space to experiment with various dynamics and scenarios.

- **Increased Arousal:** The thrill of stepping into a new role can amplify arousal, leading to a more intense and satisfying experience.

- **Personal Growth:** Engaging in role-play can foster self-discovery and personal growth, as you confront and embrace different aspects of your sexuality.

Identifying Your Roles

When developing characters for solo breeding, consider the following categories of roles:

- **The Dominant:** This character takes control, guiding the scene with confidence and authority. They embody assertiveness, using verbal and physical cues to enhance the experience.

- **The Submissive:** This role embraces vulnerability and surrender, finding pleasure in relinquishing control. The submissive character may explore feelings of trust and intimacy as they engage in the breeding scene.

- **The Caregiver:** This character focuses on nurturing and emotional connection, creating a safe and loving environment for breeding. They may emphasize aftercare and emotional bonding throughout the scene.

- **The Adventurer:** This role seeks excitement and spontaneity, often incorporating elements of risk or public scenarios into their breeding experiences. The adventurer thrives on the thrill of the unknown.

- **The Fantasy Character:** Drawing inspiration from literature, film, or mythology, this character allows you to embody someone entirely different, enhancing the escapism of the breeding experience.

Practical Examples of Role Development

To illustrate how to effectively develop roles for solo breeding, consider the following scenarios:

Scenario 1: The Dominant Breeder In this scenario, you assume the role of a dominant figure, perhaps a powerful CEO or a commanding military officer. You set the scene by dressing in attire that reflects your character, such as a tailored suit or military uniform. As you engage in solo breeding, use assertive language and commands, guiding yourself through the experience with confidence. Incorporate props like a blindfold or restraints to enhance the dominant-submissive dynamic.

Scenario 2: The Submissive Lover In this scenario, you take on the role of a willing submissive, eager to please your partner (even if they are a figment of your imagination). Create an intimate setting, perhaps with soft lighting and sensual music. As you engage in solo breeding, focus on surrendering control, allowing your desires to guide the experience. Use affirmations and self-talk to reinforce your submission, heightening the emotional connection to the scene.

Scenario 3: The Adventurous Explorer For this role, imagine yourself as an adventurous character, perhaps a daring archaeologist or a bold traveler. Set the stage by incorporating elements of risk, such as engaging in solo breeding in a secluded outdoor location or a private space that feels slightly forbidden. Embrace the thrill of the unknown, allowing the excitement of your character to drive the experience.

Incorporating Props and Accessories

Utilizing props and accessories can further enhance your role-playing experience. Consider incorporating items that align with your character, such as:

- **Costumes:** Dress in attire that reflects your chosen role, whether it be a suit, lingerie, or fantasy-themed clothing.

- **Toys:** Use sexual accessories that complement your character's persona, such as restraints for the dominant role or sensual massage tools for the caregiver.

- **Setting Enhancements:** Create an environment that aligns with your character's narrative, using decor, lighting, and music to immerse yourself in the scene.

Navigating Challenges in Role-Playing

While role-playing can be immensely rewarding, it may also present challenges. Here are some common issues and strategies to navigate them:

- **Difficulty Immersing:** If you struggle to fully embody your character, try journaling about their backstory or motivations beforehand. This can help you connect with the role more deeply.

- **Self-Judgment:** It's common to feel self-conscious when engaging in solo breeding. Remind yourself that this is a personal exploration, and there is no right or wrong way to engage in role-play.

- **Balancing Fantasy and Reality:** While exploring fantasies is liberating, it's essential to maintain a clear distinction between role-play and real-life dynamics. Ensure that your experiences remain consensual and respectful of all parties involved, even in solo scenarios.

Conclusion

Developing different roles and characters for solo breeding can enhance your experience, providing a rich tapestry of fantasies to explore. By embracing the psychological benefits of role-play, identifying your desired roles, and incorporating props and accessories, you can create deeply satisfying and pleasurable solo breeding experiences. Remember to approach this exploration with an open mind and a spirit of adventure, allowing your fantasies to unfold in new and exciting ways.

Creating a Sense of Connection and Intimacy even in Solo Breeding

In the realm of erotic exploration, the concept of solo breeding may initially seem paradoxical. How can one cultivate connection and intimacy when engaging in an act that is, by definition, solitary? Yet, the truth is that solo breeding can be a deeply personal and fulfilling experience, allowing individuals to explore their desires, fantasies, and ultimately, their connection to themselves. This section will delve into the various methods and theories that can enhance the sense of intimacy during solo breeding, providing practical strategies for achieving a deeper emotional connection.

Understanding Intimacy in Solo Breeding

Intimacy is often perceived as a shared experience between partners, characterized by emotional closeness and vulnerability. However, intimacy can also be cultivated within oneself. According to [?], self-intimacy involves recognizing and embracing one's own desires, needs, and emotions. This self-awareness is crucial in the context of solo breeding, as it allows individuals to engage with their fantasies authentically and without judgment.

The Role of Fantasy and Imagination

One of the most powerful tools for creating a sense of connection during solo breeding is the use of fantasy and imagination. Engaging in vivid mental imagery can transport the individual into a world where they feel desired and connected. Research by [?] suggests that individuals who actively employ fantasy during sexual experiences report higher levels of satisfaction and emotional fulfillment.

To harness the power of fantasy, consider the following techniques:

- **Visualization:** Create a detailed mental scenario that encompasses your breeding desires. Imagine the sights, sounds, and sensations that would accompany this experience. This can include visualizing a partner, the environment, and the emotions you would feel.

- **Erotic Journaling:** Writing down your fantasies can serve as a powerful tool for self-exploration. Describe your ideal breeding scene in detail, allowing yourself to immerse in the emotions and sensations associated with it.

- **Guided Meditation:** Utilize guided meditations specifically designed to enhance erotic experiences. These can help you focus your mind and create a deeper sense of connection with your desires.

Incorporating Sensory Elements

The senses play a crucial role in creating an intimate atmosphere during solo breeding. Engaging multiple senses can enhance arousal and deepen the connection to oneself. Consider the following sensory elements:

- **Aromatherapy:** Use essential oils or scented candles to create a sensual atmosphere. Scents such as jasmine, sandalwood, or vanilla can evoke feelings of warmth and intimacy.

- **Music:** Curate a playlist of erotic or romantic music that resonates with your fantasies. The right soundtrack can elevate your mood and enhance the emotional connection to your solo experience.

- **Textures:** Incorporate various textures into your environment. Soft fabrics, silk sheets, or even body-safe materials can heighten tactile sensations and create a more immersive experience.

Mindfulness and Presence

Practicing mindfulness during solo breeding can foster a profound sense of connection and intimacy with oneself. Mindfulness involves being fully present in the moment, allowing you to experience your desires without distraction or judgment. Techniques include:

- **Breath Awareness:** Focus on your breath, allowing it to guide you into a state of relaxation and presence. As you breathe deeply, visualize your desires manifesting in the moment.

- **Body Scanning:** Conduct a body scan to connect with the sensations in each part of your body. This practice helps cultivate awareness of your physical self and enhances the overall experience.

- **Non-Judgmental Observation:** Allow yourself to observe your thoughts and feelings without judgment. This can help you embrace your desires and fantasies without shame, fostering a deeper sense of intimacy.

Using Props and Accessories

Incorporating props and accessories into solo breeding can enhance the sense of connection and intimacy. These tools can serve as extensions of your desires, creating a more immersive experience. Consider the following options:

- **Sex Toys:** Explore the use of sex toys designed for solo breeding, such as vibrators or dildos. These can help simulate the sensations of multiple partners and enhance pleasure.

- **Costumes or Lingerie:** Wearing outfits that align with your breeding fantasies can create a sense of role-play, allowing you to embody your desires fully.

- **Visual Aids:** Consider using erotic literature or visual media that resonates with your breeding fantasies. This can provide inspiration and enhance the emotional connection to your experience.

Emotional Aftercare and Reflection

After engaging in solo breeding, it is essential to practice emotional aftercare. This involves taking time to reflect on the experience and process any emotions that may arise. Techniques include:

- **Journaling:** Write about your experience, focusing on the emotions and sensations you felt. This can help you integrate the experience and foster a deeper understanding of your desires.

- **Self-Care Rituals:** Engage in self-care practices that promote relaxation and emotional well-being. This can include taking a warm bath, meditating, or enjoying a favorite snack.

- **Connecting with Community:** Consider discussing your experiences with trusted friends or communities that share similar interests. This can help reinforce feelings of connection and acceptance.

In conclusion, creating a sense of connection and intimacy during solo breeding is not only possible but can be a profoundly enriching experience. By embracing self-intimacy, utilizing fantasy, engaging the senses, practicing mindfulness, incorporating props, and reflecting post-experience, individuals can cultivate a deep emotional connection with themselves. As you explore the nuances of solo breeding, remember that intimacy begins within, paving the way for a fulfilling and pleasurable journey into your desires.

Safety and Consent in Breeding Scenes

Establishing and Maintaining Consent

Communicating Boundaries and Limits

In the realm of breeding scenes, effective communication of boundaries and limits is paramount to ensure a safe and pleasurable experience for all participants involved. This section will delve into the principles of establishing boundaries, the significance of limits, and practical strategies for communicating them effectively.

Understanding Boundaries and Limits

Boundaries are personal guidelines that define what an individual is comfortable with in a given situation. They can be physical, emotional, or sexual, and they serve to protect one's well-being and autonomy. Limits, on the other hand, refer to the extent to which an individual is willing to go within those boundaries. Understanding and articulating these concepts is crucial in any erotic lifestyle, particularly in breeding scenes where the stakes of emotional and physical intimacy are heightened.

$$\text{Boundaries} = \text{Personal Comfort Zones} \qquad (18)$$

$$\text{Limits} = \text{Extent of Engagement Within Boundaries} \qquad (19)$$

The Importance of Clear Communication

Clear communication is essential for several reasons:
1. **Safety**: Establishing boundaries ensures that all participants feel safe and respected, reducing the risk of misunderstandings that could lead to emotional

or physical harm. 2. **Trust**: Open discussions about limits foster trust among participants, allowing for deeper connections and a more fulfilling experience. 3. **Pleasure**: When boundaries are respected, individuals can fully immerse themselves in the experience, enhancing pleasure and satisfaction.

Practical Strategies for Communicating Boundaries

1. Pre-Scene Discussions Before engaging in a breeding scene, it is crucial to have a candid conversation with all participants. Discussing boundaries should be an open dialogue where each person feels empowered to express their limits without fear of judgment. Questions to consider include:

- What are your hard limits (non-negotiable boundaries)? - Are there any specific activities that you are uncomfortable with? - How do you feel about physical touch, and are there areas you prefer to avoid?

2. Establishing Safe Words Safe words are an essential tool in erotic scenarios, particularly in breeding scenes where emotions can run high. A safe word is a predetermined word or phrase that participants can use to pause or stop the activity if they feel uncomfortable. It is crucial that all participants agree on a safe word before engaging in any activities.

For example, the commonly used safe words are "red" for stop and "yellow" for slow down or check-in. The importance of using a safe word lies in its ability to provide a clear and immediate signal that transcends any verbal cues that may be missed in the heat of the moment.

3. Non-Verbal Communication Signals In addition to verbal communication, non-verbal cues play a significant role in expressing boundaries. Participants should be aware of each other's body language and facial expressions. Signs of discomfort, such as tensing up, pulling away, or avoiding eye contact, should be acknowledged and addressed immediately.

Addressing Potential Problems

1. Misunderstandings Misunderstandings can arise when boundaries are not clearly communicated. For instance, one participant may assume that a certain activity is acceptable based on previous experiences, while another may view it as a hard limit. To mitigate this risk, it is essential to revisit and clarify boundaries regularly, especially if new participants join the scene.

2. **Emotional Responses** Breeding scenes can evoke intense emotional responses, which may lead to difficulty in articulating boundaries during the experience. Participants should be encouraged to check in with each other throughout the scene, allowing for adjustments to boundaries as needed. This ongoing communication can help prevent emotional distress and ensure that everyone remains comfortable.

3. **Post-Scene Reflection** Aftercare is a critical component of any breeding scene, providing an opportunity to discuss what went well and what could be improved. This reflection should include a discussion of boundaries and limits, allowing participants to express any feelings or concerns that arose during the scene.

Examples of Effective Boundary Communication

- **Example 1:** Before a breeding scene, one participant may say, "I am comfortable with oral stimulation, but I do not want to engage in anal play. Can we agree on that?"

- **Example 2:** During a breeding scene, if a participant begins to feel overwhelmed, they might use their safe word, "yellow," to signal a need for a break and check-in.

- **Example 3:** After the scene, participants might discuss, "I felt great about how we communicated during the scene, but I realized I need to set a firmer boundary about how much physical restraint I am comfortable with."

In conclusion, communicating boundaries and limits is a fundamental aspect of engaging in breeding scenes. By fostering an environment of open dialogue, establishing safe words, and being attentive to non-verbal cues, participants can create a safe and pleasurable experience that respects individual comfort zones. Regular check-ins and post-scene reflections further enhance the understanding of boundaries, ensuring that all participants feel valued and respected in their desires and limits.

Monitoring and Respecting Consent Signals

In the realm of breeding scenes, where intimacy and vulnerability intertwine, the importance of monitoring and respecting consent signals cannot be overstated. Consent is not a one-time agreement; it is an ongoing dialogue that requires active participation from all parties involved. This section delves into the theoretical underpinnings of consent signals, the challenges that may arise, and practical examples to ensure a safe and pleasurable experience.

Theoretical Framework

Consent signals can be understood through the lens of communication theory, particularly the concept of nonverbal communication. According to Mehrabian's communication model, a significant portion of our communication is nonverbal, consisting of body language, facial expressions, and tone of voice [?]. In the context of breeding scenes, these nonverbal cues can indicate comfort, excitement, hesitation, or discomfort.

The model can be summarized as follows:

$$\text{Total Communication} = 7\%\text{Words} + 38\%\text{Tone} + 55\%\text{Body Language} \quad (20)$$

This emphasizes the need for participants to be attuned to each other's signals, ensuring that consent is not merely verbal but also embodied in their interactions.

Recognizing Consent Signals

Consent signals can be categorized into verbal and nonverbal cues. Verbal consent includes clear affirmations such as "yes," "I want this," or "please continue." Nonverbal signals may include:

- **Body Language:** Open body posture, leaning in, and relaxed muscles are often indicators of enthusiasm and consent.

- **Facial Expressions:** Smiling, eye contact, and expressions of pleasure can signify consent, whereas frowning, avoiding eye contact, or grimacing may indicate discomfort.

- **Physical Touch:** Engaging in reciprocal touch, such as holding hands or caressing, can be a strong signal of consent. Conversely, pulling away or flinching should be taken seriously as a sign to pause and reassess.

It is essential to note that consent is dynamic; it can change throughout the scene. Participants must remain vigilant and responsive to these signals, ensuring that the experience remains consensual and enjoyable for everyone involved.

Challenges in Monitoring Consent Signals

Several challenges can complicate the monitoring of consent signals:

- **Ambiguity of Signals:** Nonverbal cues can sometimes be misinterpreted. For example, a participant may be shy or hesitant but still wish to proceed. Clear communication can help clarify intentions.

- **Power Dynamics:** In scenes involving power exchange, dominant partners may misread submissive partners' signals due to the inherent dynamics of control. This necessitates an explicit agreement on how consent will be monitored and respected throughout the encounter.

- **Emotional Vulnerability:** Participants may experience heightened emotions that affect their ability to communicate consent clearly. Aftercare discussions can help address any confusion or discomfort that may arise post-scene.

Practical Examples of Monitoring Consent Signals

To illustrate the importance of monitoring consent signals, consider the following scenarios:

- **Scenario 1: The Check-in Approach**
  During a breeding scene, the dominant partner pauses to check in with the submissive partner, asking, "How are you feeling? Do you want to continue?" This verbal check-in, paired with attentive observation of the submissive's body language, demonstrates respect for ongoing consent.

- **Scenario 2: The Safe Word**
  A couple has established a safe word, "red," to be used if either partner feels uncomfortable. During the scene, the submissive partner hesitates and appears tense. The dominant partner notices this change and immediately pauses, asking, "Would you like to use your safe word?" This proactive approach respects the partner's signals and reinforces the importance of consent.

- **Scenario 3: Post-Scene Debrief**
  After a breeding scene, partners engage in a debrief where they discuss what felt good and what did not. This conversation allows both partners to express any concerns or discomforts that may not have been apparent during the scene, emphasizing the need for continuous consent and communication.

Conclusion

Monitoring and respecting consent signals is crucial in breeding scenes, ensuring that all participants feel safe, valued, and engaged. By fostering an environment of open communication and attentiveness to both verbal and nonverbal cues, partners can navigate their desires and boundaries effectively. Remember, consent is an ongoing process that requires vigilance, empathy, and mutual respect. Embracing this dynamic not only enhances the experience but also deepens the connection between partners, creating a fulfilling and erotic journey together.

Navigating Emotional Boundaries

In the context of breeding scenes, emotional boundaries play a crucial role in ensuring that all participants feel safe, respected, and fulfilled. Emotional boundaries refer to the limits we set regarding our feelings and how we allow others to interact with those feelings. They help define where one person's emotional space ends and another's begins. Navigating these boundaries effectively is essential for a positive and enriching experience in breeding scenarios.

Understanding Emotional Boundaries

Emotional boundaries can be complex, as they often intersect with psychological factors such as trust, vulnerability, and past experiences. According to [?], emotional boundaries can be likened to the invisible lines we draw in our relationships, determining how much of ourselves we are willing to share and how much we want to protect. In breeding scenes, these boundaries can significantly affect the emotional dynamics between participants.

Common Problems with Emotional Boundaries

1. **Overstepping Boundaries**: One of the most common issues in breeding scenes is the unintentional overstepping of emotional boundaries. This can occur when one partner assumes that the other is comfortable with certain actions or discussions without having established clear consent. For example, discussing future breeding possibilities or expressing deep emotional attachments without prior agreement can lead to discomfort or distress.

2. **Miscommunication**: Misunderstandings regarding emotional boundaries can arise from a lack of clear communication. Participants may have different interpretations of what is acceptable, leading to feelings of betrayal or

ESTABLISHING AND MAINTAINING CONSENT

hurt. For instance, one partner might feel a strong emotional connection after a breeding scene, while the other may view it as purely physical.

3. **Fear of Vulnerability**: Engaging in breeding scenes often requires a level of vulnerability that can be intimidating. Participants may fear that exposing their emotional needs or boundaries will lead to rejection or judgment. This fear can create a barrier to open communication, making it difficult to navigate emotional landscapes effectively.

Strategies for Navigating Emotional Boundaries

To navigate emotional boundaries successfully within breeding scenes, consider the following strategies:

1. **Open Dialogue**: Establishing an open line of communication is paramount. Before engaging in breeding scenes, discuss your emotional boundaries explicitly. Use questions such as:

- What are your emotional needs during and after the scene?
- Are there any topics or actions that make you uncomfortable?
- How do you feel about the potential for emotional attachment?

This dialogue should be ongoing, allowing for adjustments as feelings evolve.

2. **Active Listening**: Practice active listening during discussions. This means fully concentrating on what your partner is saying, acknowledging their feelings, and responding thoughtfully. Techniques such as paraphrasing or summarizing what your partner has expressed can enhance understanding and demonstrate empathy.

3. **Setting Clear Boundaries**: Clearly define your emotional boundaries and encourage your partner to do the same. Use "I" statements to express your feelings without placing blame. For example:

> I feel overwhelmed when we discuss future breeding plans immediately after a scene.

4. **Regular Check-Ins**: After a breeding scene, conduct regular check-ins to discuss how each participant felt during the experience. This can help identify any areas where boundaries may have been crossed or where emotional discomfort arose. Questions to consider include:

- How did you feel during the scene?
- Were there any moments that felt uncomfortable or unexpected?

♦ What can we do differently next time to enhance our emotional safety?

5. **Establishing Safe Words**: While safe words are typically associated with physical boundaries, they can also be useful for emotional boundaries. Agree on a safe word that can be used if one partner feels emotionally overwhelmed or uncomfortable during the scene. This word should be respected immediately, allowing for a pause or reassessment of the situation.

6. **Aftercare Practices**: Aftercare is vital in breeding scenes, as it provides an opportunity to reconnect and reaffirm emotional boundaries. Engaging in aftercare practices such as cuddling, discussing the scene, or simply being present for each other can help reinforce emotional safety and intimacy.

Examples of Navigating Emotional Boundaries

Consider the following scenarios to illustrate the importance of navigating emotional boundaries:

- **Scenario 1**: During a breeding scene, one partner expresses a desire for deeper emotional connection, while the other feels overwhelmed by the intensity of the experience. By pausing the scene and discussing their feelings, they can recalibrate their boundaries and find a compromise that satisfies both parties.

- **Scenario 2**: After a breeding scene, one partner feels a surge of emotional attachment and wants to discuss future possibilities, while the other prefers to keep things casual. By having a candid conversation about their feelings and desires, they can establish a mutual understanding that respects each partner's emotional boundaries.

In conclusion, navigating emotional boundaries in breeding scenes requires intentional communication, empathy, and a commitment to mutual respect. By understanding and respecting each other's emotional landscapes, participants can create a safe and fulfilling breeding experience that enhances intimacy and connection.

Consent in Group Breeding Dynamics

In the realm of group breeding dynamics, consent becomes a multifaceted and crucial element that requires careful navigation. The complexities of multiple participants introduce layers of interaction, power dynamics, and emotional investment that can significantly impact the experience. This section explores the essential nature of consent within these contexts, addressing theoretical underpinnings, potential challenges, and practical examples to guide participants toward a fulfilling and safe experience.

Theoretical Framework of Consent

Consent, at its core, is the mutual agreement between all parties involved to engage in specific activities. In group settings, this concept expands beyond a simple yes or no; it encompasses ongoing communication, negotiation, and the ability to withdraw consent at any point. According to *The Consent Model* (Smith, 2018), consent can be understood through the following principles:

- **Informed:** All participants must have a clear understanding of what they are consenting to, including the activities involved, potential risks, and the boundaries set by each individual.

- **Freely Given:** Consent must be provided voluntarily, without coercion or manipulation. Each participant should feel empowered to express their desires and limits.

- **Reversible:** Consent is not a one-time agreement; it can be revoked at any moment. Participants should be encouraged to communicate their feelings and changes in comfort levels throughout the experience.

- **Specific:** Consent should be specific to the activities being undertaken. General consent for a group dynamic does not imply consent for all possible actions within that context.

Challenges in Group Dynamics

While the theoretical framework provides a solid foundation, several challenges may arise when navigating consent in group breeding dynamics:

- **Miscommunication:** With multiple participants, the risk of miscommunication increases. Assumptions about each other's boundaries can lead to discomfort or violation of consent. It is essential to establish clear communication channels and check in with each participant regularly.

- **Power Imbalances:** In group dynamics, certain individuals may hold more power or influence, whether due to experience, charisma, or social status. This can create pressure for others to conform to the desires of those in power, potentially compromising their own consent. Addressing power dynamics openly and ensuring that every voice is heard is vital.

- **Emotional Responses:** Engaging in breeding scenes can evoke strong emotional reactions. Participants may feel vulnerable or exposed, leading to changes in their comfort levels. It is crucial to create a supportive environment where individuals feel safe to express their feelings and withdraw consent if necessary.

Practical Strategies for Ensuring Consent

To navigate the complexities of consent in group breeding dynamics effectively, consider the following strategies:

1. **Pre-Scene Negotiation:** Before engaging in any activities, hold a meeting with all participants to discuss boundaries, desires, and limits. Use this time to establish safe words and signals that can be used if someone feels uncomfortable during the scene. This negotiation process fosters trust and ensures everyone is on the same page.

2. **Establishing Check-Ins:** During the scene, implement regular check-ins to gauge each participant's comfort level. Simple questions like, "How are you feeling?" or "Is everyone still okay with this?" can provide opportunities for participants to express any concerns without feeling pressured.

3. **Creating a Safe Environment:** Design the physical space to promote safety and comfort. This includes ensuring privacy, providing adequate space for everyone, and having a designated area for participants to withdraw if they need a break. The environment should facilitate open communication and support.

4. **Post-Scene Debriefing:** After the scene, hold a debriefing session to discuss what worked well and any challenges that arose. This provides an opportunity for participants to share their feelings and process the experience, reinforcing the importance of consent and communication.

Examples of Consent in Action

Consider the following scenarios to illustrate the application of consent principles in group breeding dynamics:

- **Scenario 1:** A group of four individuals decides to engage in a breeding scene. Before starting, they establish that everyone is comfortable with the idea of multiple loads and agree on safe words. During the scene, one participant feels overwhelmed and uses the safe word. The group immediately stops, respecting the individual's need to withdraw from the activity. This demonstrates the importance of ongoing communication and the ability to revoke consent.

- **Scenario 2:** In a larger gathering, a participant expresses interest in exploring a specific fantasy involving multiple partners. Before proceeding, they discuss their boundaries and ensure that all involved parties are comfortable with the proposed activities. As the scene unfolds, the participants check in with one another, allowing for real-time adjustments to the dynamics based on comfort levels. This proactive approach highlights the significance of pre-scene negotiation and continuous consent.

Conclusion

Consent in group breeding dynamics is not merely a checkbox to be marked but an ongoing process that requires active participation, communication, and respect for individual boundaries. By understanding the theoretical framework of consent, recognizing the challenges inherent in group dynamics, and implementing practical strategies, participants can create a safe and pleasurable environment for all involved. Ultimately, fostering a culture of consent enhances the overall experience, deepening connections and ensuring that everyone feels valued and respected in their desires and boundaries.

Consent in Public Breeding Scenes and Play Parties

In the realm of public breeding scenes and play parties, consent becomes an intricate dance, one that requires clarity, communication, and an unwavering commitment to respect. As we navigate these shared spaces of erotic exploration, it is imperative to understand the unique challenges and dynamics that arise in public settings, where the visibility of our desires can heighten both excitement and anxiety.

The Nature of Consent in Public Spaces

Consent is a foundational principle in any sexual encounter, but in public breeding scenes, it takes on additional layers of complexity. The nature of consent in these environments can be influenced by several factors:

- **Visibility:** The presence of onlookers can amplify the thrill of the scene, yet it also necessitates a heightened awareness of the boundaries established by all parties involved.

- **Group Dynamics:** In a play party, the interactions between multiple participants may create a dynamic where consent is not only about individual agreements but also about the collective understanding of the scene's limits.

- **Fluidity of Consent:** Consent can be fluid in public settings, as the atmosphere may shift from one of intimate connection to one of exhibitionism, requiring ongoing negotiation and reaffirmation of boundaries.

Establishing Consent Before the Scene

Prior to engaging in public breeding scenes, it is vital to establish consent through clear communication. Here are some strategies to ensure that all participants are on the same page:

1. **Pre-Scene Negotiation:** Engage in open discussions with all parties involved to outline desires, limits, and safe words. This conversation should occur well before the scene begins to allow for thoughtful consideration.

2. **Clear Safe Words:** Establish safe words that are easily remembered and understood. In public settings, consider using a color-coded system (e.g., green for go, yellow for slow down, red for stop) to facilitate quick communication in the heat of the moment.

3. **Consent Check-Ins:** During the scene, incorporate regular check-ins to reaffirm consent. Simple questions like "Are you okay?" or "Do you want to continue?" can help maintain a sense of safety and mutual enjoyment.

Monitoring Consent Signals

In a public breeding scene, non-verbal cues play a significant role in understanding consent. Participants should be attuned to both verbal and non-verbal signals, which can indicate comfort or discomfort. Here are some key considerations:

- **Body Language:** Pay attention to the body language of all participants. Signs of enjoyment may include relaxed posture, open body language, and enthusiastic participation. Conversely, crossed arms, tense muscles, or averted gazes may signal discomfort.

- **Vocal Cues:** Listen for vocalizations that express pleasure or distress. While moans and gasps may indicate enjoyment, sudden silences or changes in tone can be red flags.

- **Environmental Awareness:** Be mindful of the surroundings and the reactions of onlookers. The presence of an audience can influence individual comfort levels, necessitating adjustments to the scene as needed.

Navigating Emotional Boundaries

Emotional boundaries can be particularly challenging in public breeding scenes. Participants may feel vulnerable due to the exposure of their desires and bodies. To navigate these emotional landscapes:

- **Post-Scene Debriefing:** After the scene, take time to discuss the experience with all participants. This debriefing allows individuals to express their feelings, address any concerns, and reinforce the emotional connection forged during the scene.

- **Recognizing Triggers:** Be aware of potential triggers that may arise in public settings, such as unexpected attention or judgment from onlookers. Establishing a safe space for participants to express discomfort can help mitigate these challenges.

- **Support Systems:** Create a support system within the group, where participants feel comfortable reaching out to each other for reassurance and validation. This network can enhance emotional safety and foster deeper connections.

Consent in Group Breeding Dynamics

When engaging in group breeding dynamics, the complexity of consent multiplies. Here are some strategies to navigate these scenarios:

- **Collective Consent Agreements:** Prior to the scene, establish a collective agreement that outlines the dynamics of participation, including who will engage with whom and any limitations on interactions.

- **Role Assignments:** Clearly define roles within the group to avoid misunderstandings. Participants should be aware of their roles and the expectations associated with them, whether they are dominant, submissive, or observers.

- **Exit Strategies:** Ensure that all participants have a clear exit strategy if they feel uncomfortable at any point. This may involve signaling to a designated safe person or using a pre-agreed safe word.

Consent in Public Breeding Scenes: Real-World Examples

To illustrate the principles of consent in public breeding scenes, consider the following hypothetical scenarios:

- **Scenario 1: The Play Party** - At a local BDSM play party, a couple decides to explore breeding fantasies in front of a small audience. Before the scene, they communicate their desires and establish boundaries. During the performance, they frequently check in with each other, ensuring that both partners feel comfortable and excited about the unfolding activities. The audience's presence enhances their experience rather than detracting from it, as they feel supported by the shared energy of the space.

- **Scenario 2: The Public Park** - In a more adventurous setting, a group of friends decides to engage in a public breeding scene at a secluded area of a park. Prior to beginning, they establish clear consent agreements and safe words. As they engage, they remain vigilant about their surroundings, adjusting their activities as needed to maintain a sense of privacy and safety. After the scene, they gather to discuss their experiences, addressing any feelings of vulnerability or discomfort that arose during the public display.

Conclusion

In conclusion, consent in public breeding scenes and play parties is a multifaceted and dynamic aspect of the erotic lifestyle. By prioritizing clear communication, monitoring consent signals, and navigating emotional boundaries, participants can create a safe and exhilarating environment for exploration. Embracing the thrill of public encounters while respecting the autonomy and comfort of all involved enhances the experience, fostering deeper connections and shared satisfaction. As we continue to explore the boundaries of our desires, let us remain committed to the principles of consent that guide our journeys in the world of eroticism.

Exploring Power Dynamics in Breeding Scenes

Dominance and Submission

Understanding Power Exchange

Power exchange is a fundamental concept in the realm of BDSM and erotic lifestyles, particularly within breeding scenes. It refers to the dynamic relationship between individuals where one person voluntarily relinquishes control to another. This exchange of power can create an exhilarating atmosphere of trust, vulnerability, and heightened intimacy, allowing participants to explore their desires and fantasies more deeply.

Theoretical Framework

The theory of power exchange is rooted in the principles of dominance and submission. According to [?], power dynamics can be understood through the lens of social and psychological constructs that govern interpersonal relationships. The dynamics often manifest in various forms, including:

- **Dominance:** The act of exerting control or authority over another individual. This may involve setting rules, directing actions, or making decisions on behalf of the submissive partner.

- **Submission:** The willingness to yield control to another individual. This often involves trust and a desire to explore vulnerability in a safe and consensual environment.

- **Negotiation:** The process by which participants discuss and agree upon the terms of their power exchange. Effective negotiation is crucial for establishing boundaries, limits, and safe words.

Psychological Aspects

The psychological underpinnings of power exchange can be traced to several key concepts:

1. **Trust:** A cornerstone of any power exchange dynamic, trust allows the submissive partner to feel safe in surrendering control. The dominant partner must be aware of their responsibility to uphold this trust.

2. **Vulnerability:** Engaging in power exchange often requires both partners to confront their vulnerabilities. The submissive partner exposes their desires and fears, while the dominant partner must navigate the responsibility that comes with their power.

3. **Aftercare:** Post-scene care is essential in power exchange relationships. It provides an opportunity for both partners to reconnect, process their experiences, and reaffirm their bond.

Common Challenges

Despite its allure, power exchange can present challenges that require careful consideration:

- **Miscommunication:** A lack of clear communication can lead to misunderstandings about boundaries and expectations. It is vital to engage in open dialogues before and after scenes to ensure both partners are aligned.

- **Emotional Risks:** Power exchange can evoke strong emotions, including feelings of inadequacy or insecurity. Participants should be prepared to navigate these emotions and seek support if needed.

- **Societal Stigma:** Engaging in power exchange dynamics may invite judgment from those outside the community. Partners should be equipped to discuss their choices with others if they choose to do so.

Examples of Power Exchange in Breeding Scenes

To illustrate the concept of power exchange in breeding scenes, consider the following scenarios:

> **Example**
>
> Scenario 1: A couple decides to engage in a breeding scene where the dominant partner takes control of the submissive partner's pleasure. The dominant partner sets specific rules about when and how the submissive can orgasm, heightening the anticipation and intensity of the experience. This dynamic fosters trust, as the submissive partner relies on the dominant to respect their boundaries while pushing their limits.

> **Example**
>
> Scenario 2: In a group breeding setting, one participant may take on the role of the "breeder," while others assume submissive roles. The breeder establishes rules for the scene, including safe words and limits, and the submissive partners agree to follow these guidelines. This power exchange creates a shared experience that enhances the erotic atmosphere, allowing for exploration of desires in a consensual and structured manner.

Conclusion

Understanding power exchange is essential for anyone looking to explore breeding scenes within the erotic lifestyle. By recognizing the dynamics of dominance and submission, participants can foster deeper connections, enhance their experiences, and navigate the complexities of their desires safely and consensually. As power exchange unfolds, it is crucial to maintain open lines of communication, prioritize trust, and engage in aftercare to ensure a fulfilling and enriching experience for all involved.

Incorporating BDSM Elements into Breeding Scenes

Breeding scenes, characterized by their intimate and primal nature, can be significantly enhanced through the incorporation of BDSM elements. This fusion not only adds layers of complexity and excitement but also deepens the emotional and psychological connections between participants. In this section, we will explore how to effectively blend BDSM with breeding scenes, addressing key theories, potential challenges, and practical examples.

Theoretical Foundations of BDSM in Breeding

BDSM, which stands for Bondage, Discipline, Dominance, Submission, Sadism, and Masochism, operates on the principles of power exchange, consent, and trust. When integrated into breeding scenes, these principles can amplify the intensity of the experience.

The **power dynamics** inherent in BDSM allow participants to explore their desires in a structured environment. For example, a dominant partner may take control during a breeding scene, dictating the pace and intensity, which can heighten arousal and anticipation for the submissive partner. This dynamic can create a fertile ground for exploring themes of surrender and vulnerability, which are often central to breeding fantasies.

Challenges in Blending BDSM and Breeding

While the incorporation of BDSM elements can enhance breeding scenes, it is essential to recognize and address potential challenges:

- **Consent and Communication:** Clear and ongoing communication is vital in BDSM practices. Establishing safe words and boundaries is crucial, especially in breeding scenarios where emotions can run high. Participants should engage in thorough discussions about their limits and desires before the scene begins.

- **Emotional Aftercare:** BDSM often requires aftercare to help participants process their experiences. In breeding scenes, the emotional weight can be significant. It is important to have a plan for aftercare that addresses both physical and emotional needs, ensuring that all parties feel safe and supported post-scene.

- **Health and Safety Considerations:** Breeding scenes may involve risks related to sexual health. Incorporating BDSM elements, such as bondage, can complicate these considerations. Participants must prioritize safety and hygiene, discussing any health concerns openly before engaging in activities.

Practical Examples of Incorporating BDSM into Breeding Scenes

To effectively blend BDSM with breeding scenes, consider the following practical examples:

- **Bondage Techniques:** Use bondage to enhance the feeling of surrender. For instance, binding a partner's hands can create a sense of helplessness that intensifies the breeding fantasy. Consider using soft restraints, such as silk ties or cuffs, to ensure comfort while still maintaining control.

- **Roleplay Scenarios:** Engage in roleplay that incorporates power dynamics. For example, one partner could take on the role of a "breeder" while the other is a "submissive." This dynamic can heighten the intensity of the breeding scene, allowing for exploration of dominance and submission.

- **Sensory Deprivation:** Introduce elements of sensory deprivation, such as blindfolds or earplugs, to enhance the experience. By limiting one sense, the remaining senses become more acute, intensifying the sensations experienced during the breeding scene.

- **Impact Play:** Consider incorporating light impact play, such as spanking or flogging, to build arousal and excitement. The physical sensations can serve as a prelude to the breeding act, creating a heightened state of anticipation.

- **Verbal Domination:** Use dirty talk and verbal commands to assert control. Phrases that emphasize the breeding fantasy can enhance the experience, such as "You will take all of me" or "You were made for this." The use of language can be a powerful tool in establishing dominance and enhancing pleasure.

Conclusion

Incorporating BDSM elements into breeding scenes offers a unique opportunity to deepen the emotional and physical connection between partners. By understanding the theoretical foundations, addressing potential challenges, and employing practical techniques, participants can create a rich and fulfilling experience. As with any sexual exploration, the keys to success lie in open communication, consent, and a commitment to safety. By embracing these principles, individuals can elevate their breeding scenes to new heights of pleasure and intimacy.

Negotiating Power Dynamics Safely

Negotiating power dynamics within breeding scenes requires a careful and thoughtful approach to ensure that all participants feel safe, respected, and fulfilled. Power exchange can be an exhilarating aspect of erotic play, but it also carries inherent risks that must be managed effectively. This section will explore strategies for negotiating power dynamics safely, emphasizing the importance of communication, consent, and ongoing assessment.

Understanding Power Dynamics

Power dynamics refer to the ways in which control, authority, and influence are distributed among participants in a scene. In breeding scenarios, one partner may assume a dominant role while the other takes on a submissive role. This dynamic can enhance the erotic experience, allowing for deeper emotional connections and heightened pleasure. However, it is crucial to recognize that power dynamics should always be consensual and negotiated prior to engaging in any activities.

The Role of Communication

Effective communication is the cornerstone of safe power dynamics. Before engaging in breeding scenes that involve power exchange, all participants should engage in open and honest discussions about their desires, limits, and expectations. This conversation should cover several key areas:

- **Desires and Fantasies:** Each participant should express what they hope to achieve from the scene. This includes discussing specific breeding fantasies, desires for submission or dominance, and any particular scenarios they wish to explore.

- **Limits and Boundaries:** Establishing hard and soft limits is essential. Hard limits are activities that are off-limits under any circumstances, while soft limits may be negotiable depending on the context. For example, a participant may have a hard limit against certain types of physical restraint but may be open to exploring light bondage.

- **Safe Words:** Agree on safe words or signals that can be used to pause or stop the scene. Commonly used safe words include "red" for stop and "yellow" for slow down or check-in. These words should be respected without question, ensuring that all participants feel secure in their ability to communicate discomfort or the need for a break.

DOMINANCE AND SUBMISSION

- **Aftercare:** Discussing aftercare needs is vital for emotional well-being post-scene. Aftercare can involve physical comfort, emotional support, and reassurance, which are particularly important in power exchange dynamics. Each participant should express their aftercare preferences, which may include cuddling, verbal affirmations, or quiet time alone.

Consent and Ongoing Assessment

Consent is not a one-time agreement; it is an ongoing process that should be revisited throughout the scene. Participants should regularly check in with each other to ensure that everyone remains comfortable and engaged. This can be achieved through verbal check-ins or non-verbal cues, depending on the dynamics established.

$$C(t) = C_0 + \int_0^t \frac{dC}{dt} dt \qquad (21)$$

Where: - $C(t)$ represents the current state of consent at time t, - C_0 is the initial agreement reached before the scene, - $\frac{dC}{dt}$ is the rate of change in consent during the scene.

This equation illustrates that consent can evolve over time, and it is the responsibility of all participants to ensure that it is maintained throughout the experience.

Addressing Potential Problems

Despite thorough preparation, issues may arise during a breeding scene involving power dynamics. It is essential to be prepared for potential problems and have strategies in place to address them:

- **Miscommunication:** Misunderstandings can occur, leading to discomfort or distress. If a participant feels that their limits are being pushed, they should feel empowered to use their safe word or signal. It is crucial for the dominant partner to respect this immediately and pause the scene.

- **Emotional Triggers:** Power dynamics can evoke strong emotional responses. Participants should be aware of their triggers and communicate them beforehand. If an emotional trigger arises during the scene, taking a break to address it is vital.

- **Physical Safety:** Ensure that all activities are conducted with physical safety in mind. This includes using safe equipment, being aware of the physical limits of each participant, and having a first aid kit readily available in case of accidents.

Examples of Safe Negotiation in Breeding Scenes

To illustrate safe negotiation practices, consider the following scenarios:

- **Scenario 1:** A couple discusses their interest in a breeding scene where one partner desires to take on a dominant role. They agree to establish a safe word and discuss what specific actions will take place, such as verbal commands and physical restraint. Throughout the scene, they check in with each other to ensure mutual comfort.

- **Scenario 2:** In a group breeding setting, participants engage in a pre-scene meeting to outline their limits and desires. They establish a group safe word and agree on how to handle any discomfort that may arise. During the scene, they maintain open communication, allowing for adjustments as necessary.

In conclusion, negotiating power dynamics safely in breeding scenes requires a commitment to communication, consent, and continuous assessment. By fostering an environment of trust and respect, participants can explore the thrilling aspects of power exchange while ensuring that their experiences are safe and fulfilling. The key to successful power dynamics lies in the collaborative effort of all involved, creating a shared space for exploration and connection.

Exploring Dominance and Submission Roles in Breeding

The exploration of dominance and submission (D/s) roles within breeding scenes adds a profound layer of complexity and richness to the experience. Understanding these dynamics is essential for those interested in integrating power exchange into their breeding fantasies. This section will delve into the theoretical underpinnings of D/s relationships, common problems that may arise, and practical examples to illustrate the nuances involved.

Theoretical Framework of Dominance and Submission

At its core, the D/s dynamic is characterized by an exchange of power, where one partner (the Dominant) takes control, while the other (the submissive) relinquishes

DOMINANCE AND SUBMISSION

it. This relationship can manifest in various forms, from casual encounters to deeply committed partnerships. The power exchange is consensual and often negotiated, creating a safe space for both parties to explore their desires.

The psychological aspects of D/s dynamics can be examined through the lens of *Erikson's stages of psychosocial development*, particularly the stages of intimacy vs. isolation and generativity vs. stagnation. In a breeding context, the act of submission can foster intimacy, allowing the submissive partner to explore vulnerability and trust, while the Dominant partner may experience a sense of generativity, nurturing and guiding the submissive through the experience.

Common Challenges in D/s Breeding Scenarios

While the D/s dynamic can enhance breeding scenes, several challenges may arise:

- **Miscommunication:** A lack of clear communication regarding desires, boundaries, and safe words can lead to misunderstandings and discomfort. It is vital to establish open lines of communication before engaging in breeding activities.

- **Consent Issues:** Consent must be explicit and ongoing. Partners should regularly check in with each other to ensure that both parties feel comfortable and safe throughout the experience.

- **Emotional Aftermath:** The intense nature of D/s dynamics can lead to emotional vulnerability. Aftercare is crucial to address any feelings that may arise post-scene and to reaffirm the connection between partners.

Examples of D/s Roles in Breeding Scenes

To illustrate the D/s dynamic in breeding, consider the following scenarios:

1. **The Nurturing Dominant:** In this scenario, the Dominant partner takes on a nurturing role, guiding the submissive through the breeding experience. The Dominant may set the pace, deciding when to engage in sexual activity, and how many loads to deliver. This role can enhance the feeling of safety for the submissive, allowing them to surrender fully to the experience.

2. **The Obedient Submissive:** Here, the submissive partner embraces their role by eagerly following the Dominant's instructions. They may be tasked with specific actions, such as preparing the breeding space or engaging in

self-pleasure while awaiting the Dominant's arrival. This can heighten anticipation and enhance the overall experience.

3. **Role Reversal:** In some cases, partners may choose to switch roles, allowing both individuals to experience the dynamics of dominance and submission. This can be particularly enriching in breeding scenarios, as it fosters empathy and understanding between partners.

Incorporating BDSM Elements into Breeding Scenes

Integrating BDSM elements into breeding scenes can further enhance the D/s dynamic. Consider the following techniques:

- **Bondage:** Light bondage can be used to heighten the submissive's sense of surrender. Restraints can limit movement, intensifying the experience of being bred.

- **Impact Play:** Incorporating elements of impact play, such as spanking or flogging, can serve to heighten arousal and reinforce the power exchange.

- **Sensory Deprivation:** Blindfolds or earplugs can enhance the submissive's focus on the sensations of breeding, amplifying their experience of pleasure.

Negotiating Power Dynamics Safely

Establishing a safe environment for exploring D/s dynamics is paramount. Consider the following strategies:

- **Pre-Scene Negotiation:** Engage in thorough discussions about desires, boundaries, and safe words before the scene begins. This ensures that both partners are on the same page and can enjoy the experience without anxiety.

- **Ongoing Consent:** Regularly check in with each other during the scene to confirm that both parties are comfortable and enjoying the experience. This can be done through verbal communication or non-verbal cues.

- **Aftercare:** Aftercare is crucial in D/s dynamics, particularly in breeding scenes. Spend time together after the experience to process emotions, provide comfort, and reinforce the bond between partners.

Developing a Personal Power Dynamic in Your Breeding Lifestyle

Each couple's D/s dynamic will be unique, shaped by individual preferences and boundaries. To cultivate a fulfilling power dynamic within breeding scenes, consider the following:

- **Explore Fantasies:** Discuss and explore personal fantasies related to dominance and submission within the context of breeding. This can help partners discover new aspects of their desires.

- **Experiment with Roles:** Be open to experimenting with different roles and dynamics. This exploration can lead to deeper understanding and satisfaction within the relationship.

- **Reflect on Experiences:** After engaging in breeding scenes, take time to reflect on the experience together. Discuss what worked well and what could be improved, fostering growth in the relationship.

In conclusion, the exploration of dominance and submission roles in breeding scenes can significantly enhance the experience for both partners. By fostering open communication, understanding the psychological aspects of D/s dynamics, and incorporating BDSM elements thoughtfully, couples can create a deeply satisfying and intimate breeding experience that resonates with their desires and fantasies.

Developing a Personal Power Dynamic in Your Breeding Lifestyle

In the exploration of breeding scenes, the interplay of power dynamics can significantly enhance the experience, introducing layers of emotional and psychological engagement that deepen the connection between partners. Understanding how to develop a personal power dynamic tailored to your desires and boundaries is crucial for creating fulfilling and consensual breeding experiences.

Understanding Personal Power Dynamics

Personal power dynamics refer to the specific ways in which individuals express and negotiate power within their relationships. In the context of breeding, this dynamic can manifest through various roles, such as dominant and submissive, or even in more nuanced ways that incorporate elements of nurturing, control, and vulnerability.

The foundation of any power dynamic lies in the understanding of the following key concepts:

- **Power Exchange:** This is the process by which partners willingly give and receive power. In breeding scenes, the dominant partner may take control over the scene, while the submissive partner may surrender to the experience, creating a reciprocal exchange that heightens arousal and intimacy.

- **Role Fluidity:** Personal power dynamics are not static; they can shift and evolve. Partners may choose to alternate roles, exploring both dominance and submission, or they may establish consistent roles that resonate with their desires.

- **Emotional Safety:** Establishing a safe space for exploring power dynamics is essential. This involves clear communication about limits, desires, and aftercare, ensuring that both partners feel secure in their roles and can express their needs openly.

Theoretical Frameworks

Several theoretical frameworks can help in understanding and developing personal power dynamics within breeding lifestyles:

- **The BDSM Framework:** BDSM (Bondage, Discipline, Dominance, Submission, Sadism, and Masochism) provides a rich context for exploring power dynamics. Within this framework, the concept of *consensual non-consent* allows partners to engage in scenes that may involve elements of control and submission while maintaining a foundation of trust and consent.

- **Attachment Theory:** Understanding your attachment style can also inform your power dynamics. For instance, those with a secure attachment may feel comfortable exploring vulnerability, while those with anxious or avoidant attachments may approach power dynamics with caution. Recognizing these patterns can help partners navigate their dynamics more effectively.

- **Transactional Analysis:** This psychological theory analyzes the interactions between individuals based on three ego states: Parent, Adult, and Child. In breeding dynamics, partners may embody different ego states, influencing how they express power and negotiate roles. For example, a dominant partner may adopt a nurturing Parent role, while a submissive partner may embrace a playful Child role.

Identifying Your Personal Dynamic

Developing a personal power dynamic begins with self-reflection and communication. Here are steps to help you identify and cultivate your unique dynamic:

1. **Self-Assessment:** Take time to reflect on your desires, boundaries, and comfort levels with power exchange. Consider journaling your thoughts or discussing them with a trusted partner. Questions to ponder include:

   - What aspects of power exchange excite me?
   - Do I prefer to take control, or do I feel more comfortable surrendering?
   - How do I feel about vulnerability in intimate settings?

2. **Open Dialogue:** Engage in candid conversations with your partner about your findings. Discuss your interests in power dynamics, any fantasies you wish to explore, and establish a mutual understanding of each other's boundaries. Use this dialogue to negotiate roles and expectations, ensuring that both partners feel heard and respected.

3. **Role Play and Experimentation:** Begin exploring your dynamic through role play. This can be as simple as adopting specific titles (e.g., "Daddy" and "little one") or as elaborate as creating scenarios that encapsulate your power exchange. Experimentation allows you to test the waters of your dynamic, providing insights into what resonates with you both.

4. **Feedback and Adjustment:** After engaging in power dynamics, debrief with your partner. Discuss what worked, what didn't, and how you both felt during the experience. This feedback loop is essential for refining your dynamic and ensuring that both partners feel fulfilled and satisfied.

5. **Continuous Learning:** Power dynamics are an evolving journey. Stay open to learning about yourself and your partner as you explore new avenues of your breeding lifestyle. Attend workshops, read literature, or join communities focused on power dynamics to broaden your understanding and skills.

Examples of Personal Power Dynamics in Breeding

To illustrate the development of personal power dynamics in breeding, consider the following examples:

- **The Nurturing Dominant:** In this dynamic, one partner assumes a dominant role characterized by care and protection. They may guide the submissive partner through the breeding experience, emphasizing the emotional and physical connection. This dynamic can foster a sense of safety and trust, allowing the submissive to explore their desires fully.

- **The Playful Submissive:** Here, the submissive partner embraces a playful, mischievous role. They may tease the dominant partner, creating a lighthearted atmosphere that enhances the breeding experience. This dynamic encourages spontaneity and creativity, allowing both partners to enjoy the process without the weight of seriousness.

- **The Role Reversal:** In this scenario, partners may switch roles during a breeding session, allowing each to experience dominance and submission. This fluidity can deepen their connection, as they gain insight into each other's desires and boundaries, enhancing empathy and understanding.

Conclusion

Developing a personal power dynamic in your breeding lifestyle is a journey of exploration and self-discovery. By understanding the theoretical frameworks, engaging in self-assessment, and fostering open communication, you can create a dynamic that resonates with both you and your partner. Embrace the fluidity of roles, remain open to experimentation, and prioritize emotional safety to cultivate a breeding experience that is both fulfilling and enriching. As you navigate this landscape, remember that the ultimate goal is to enhance intimacy and pleasure, allowing your desires to flourish within the context of trust and consent.

Beyond the Bedroom: Breeding in Public and Group Settings

Public Breeding Scenes

Legal and Ethical Considerations

In the realm of breeding scenes, particularly those that occur in public or group settings, it is imperative to navigate the complex landscape of legal and ethical considerations. Engaging in such activities requires a thorough understanding of the laws governing sexual conduct in various jurisdictions, as well as a commitment to ethical practices that respect the autonomy and rights of all participants involved.

Understanding Local Laws

The first step in ensuring a safe and consensual breeding experience in public spaces is to familiarize oneself with the legal framework surrounding sexual activities in those areas. Laws can vary significantly from one location to another, and what may be permissible in one jurisdiction could be deemed illegal in another.

- **Public Decency Laws:** Many regions have laws prohibiting public indecency, which can include sexual acts performed in view of the public. Engaging in breeding scenes in public settings may attract legal repercussions if such acts are considered indecent.

- **Age of Consent:** It is crucial to ensure that all participants are of legal age and capable of giving informed consent. Engaging with individuals below the age of consent can lead to severe legal consequences, including criminal charges.

- **Permits and Permissions:** Some public spaces may require permits for any organized gatherings or events that involve sexual activities. It is advisable to check with local authorities or venue management to ensure compliance with any necessary regulations.

Ethical Considerations

Beyond legalities, ethical considerations play a vital role in fostering a respectful and consensual environment for breeding scenes. Ethical practices ensure that all participants feel safe, valued, and empowered throughout their experience.

- **Informed Consent:** Consent must be informed, enthusiastic, and ongoing. Participants should be fully aware of what the breeding scene entails, including potential risks and the nature of the activities involved. It is essential to discuss boundaries and safe words, ensuring that everyone has the right to withdraw consent at any time without fear of repercussion.

- **Respect for Privacy:** Engaging in public breeding scenes can blur the lines of privacy. Participants should be mindful of the presence of bystanders and consider how their actions may affect others. It is important to establish clear boundaries regarding what can be shared publicly about the experience and to respect the anonymity of all involved.

- **Community Standards:** Different communities have varying standards regarding acceptable behavior. It is vital to gauge the comfort levels of both participants and observers, ensuring that the breeding scene does not infringe upon the rights or comfort of others. Engaging with local communities and understanding their norms can help in making informed decisions about where and how to conduct breeding scenes.

Case Studies and Examples

To illustrate the importance of understanding legal and ethical considerations, consider the following hypothetical scenarios:

1. **Scenario 1: Public Park Gathering**
   A group of individuals decides to organize a breeding scene in a public park. They have not consulted local laws regarding public indecency. As the scene unfolds, park authorities intervene, leading to legal consequences for the participants. This scenario underscores the necessity of researching local laws before engaging in public activities.

2. Scenario 2: Consent Violation
   In a group setting, one participant attempts to engage another without explicit consent, assuming that the atmosphere allows for such behavior. This leads to discomfort and feelings of violation for the non-consenting individual. This example highlights the critical importance of establishing clear communication and consent protocols before any breeding scene.

3. Scenario 3: Respecting Bystanders
   A couple engages in a breeding scene at a public event, unaware of the discomfort it may cause to nearby families. Several attendees express their discontent, leading to a negative response from event organizers. This situation illustrates the need to consider the broader community and respect the comfort levels of others when planning public activities.

Conclusion

Navigating the legal and ethical considerations of breeding scenes in public and group settings is paramount for creating a safe and enjoyable experience for all participants. By understanding local laws, prioritizing informed consent, and respecting community standards, individuals can foster an environment that honors the desires and boundaries of everyone involved. Engaging in open dialogues about these considerations not only enhances personal experiences but also contributes to a more informed and responsible breeding community.

Finding Safe and Consensual Public Spaces

Finding safe and consensual public spaces for breeding scenes is a vital aspect of exploring this thrilling facet of the erotic lifestyle. The allure of public settings can heighten arousal, but it also requires careful consideration of legal, ethical, and safety factors. This section will guide you through the process of identifying appropriate venues, ensuring consent, and navigating the complexities of public breeding dynamics.

Understanding the Landscape of Public Spaces

Public spaces can range from private venues that allow for group gatherings to more open environments like parks, beaches, or even clubs. The key to a successful public breeding scene lies in understanding the nature of the space you choose.

- **Private Venues:** These include rented rooms, hotels, or clubs that cater to adult activities. They often provide a controlled environment with fewer legal concerns.

- **Open Public Spaces:** Parks, beaches, and other outdoor settings can offer a sense of thrill but come with increased risks, including legal repercussions and potential interruptions.

Legal and Ethical Considerations

Before engaging in any public breeding scene, it is crucial to familiarize yourself with local laws regarding public decency and sexual conduct. Engaging in sexual acts in public can lead to serious legal consequences, including arrest or fines.

$$\text{Legal Risk} = f(\text{Location}, \text{Activity}, \text{Visibility}) \qquad (22)$$

Where: - **Location** refers to the legal status of sexual activity in that area. - **Activity** refers to the nature of the acts performed. - **Visibility** refers to how exposed the participants are to the public eye.

This equation illustrates that the legal risk increases with more visible and explicit activities in locations where public sexual conduct is prohibited.

Finding the Right Spaces

To locate suitable public spaces, consider the following strategies:

- **Community Events:** Look for adult-friendly events, such as sex-positive festivals, parties, or gatherings that promote alternative lifestyles. These environments often foster a sense of community and shared interests.

- **Social Media and Online Forums:** Engage with communities on platforms dedicated to alternative lifestyles. Members often share recommendations for safe venues, tips, and experiences.

- **Adult Clubs and Parties:** Many cities have clubs specifically designed for adult entertainment. These venues typically have established rules and guidelines that promote safety and consent.

Negotiating Boundaries and Privacy

Once you identify a potential public space, it is essential to negotiate boundaries and privacy with your partners. This includes:

- **Establishing Safe Words:** Agree on a safe word or signal that can be used to pause or stop the scene if necessary.

- **Discussing Visibility:** Consider how visible you want to be during the scene. Some may prefer to be more discreet, while others may enjoy the thrill of being seen.

- **Planning for Interruptions:** Have a plan in place for what to do if someone approaches or if you feel uncomfortable. This could involve moving to a more secluded area or stopping the activity altogether.

Building Community and Connection

Public breeding scenes can foster a sense of community and connection among participants. Engaging in these activities in a consensual and safe manner can lead to shared experiences and deeper relationships.

- **Creating a Support Network:** Establish connections with like-minded individuals who share your interests. This can enhance your experiences and provide a support system for navigating public dynamics.

- **Participating in Group Activities:** Join group outings or events that focus on erotic exploration. These gatherings often provide a safe space to experiment and connect with others.

Conclusion

Finding safe and consensual public spaces for breeding scenes requires careful planning, communication, and awareness of legal and ethical considerations. By understanding the landscape of public spaces, negotiating boundaries, and building community connections, you can enhance your breeding experiences while ensuring safety and consent. Remember, the thrill of public breeding lies not just in the act itself, but in the shared journey of exploration and discovery with your partners.

Maximizing Pleasure in Public Settings

Public breeding scenes can create an exhilarating blend of thrill and intimacy, but they require careful planning and consideration to ensure that pleasure is maximized for all participants. This section will explore various strategies to enhance enjoyment while maintaining safety and consent in public environments.

Understanding the Public Setting

When engaging in public breeding scenes, it is essential to understand the dynamics of the environment. Public spaces can range from secluded parks to bustling clubs, each presenting unique opportunities and challenges. The thrill of being observed can heighten arousal, but it is crucial to navigate the space with respect for others and awareness of legal boundaries.

Choosing the Right Location

Selecting an appropriate location is paramount. Consider the following factors when choosing your public setting:

- **Privacy:** Look for areas that offer a degree of seclusion, such as a quiet corner of a park or a private room in a club. The goal is to minimize the risk of unwanted attention while still allowing for a sense of exposure.

- **Ambiance:** The atmosphere can significantly impact the experience. Choose locations that evoke a sensual vibe—think dim lighting, soft music, or natural surroundings that enhance the mood.

- **Accessibility:** Ensure that the location is easily accessible for all participants. Consider mobility issues and the comfort of everyone involved.

Negotiating Boundaries and Consent

Before engaging in any public scene, open communication is vital. Discuss boundaries and consent thoroughly with all participants. Use the following strategies:

- **Safe Words:** Establish clear safe words that can be used to pause or stop the scene if anyone feels uncomfortable.

- **Non-Verbal Signals:** In a public setting, verbal communication may not always be feasible. Agree on discreet non-verbal signals that can indicate comfort or the need to pause.

- **Consent Check-Ins:** Regularly check in with all participants to ensure everyone is comfortable and enjoying the experience. This can be done through subtle gestures or brief eye contact.

Enhancing Sensory Experiences

To maximize pleasure in public settings, consider incorporating sensory elements that heighten arousal and intimacy:

- **Touch:** Utilize light touches or caresses that can be easily concealed. The thrill of being discreetly intimate can amplify excitement.

- **Sound:** Whispering sweet nothings or dirty talk can create an intimate atmosphere while remaining subtle. The sound of your partner's breath or soft moans can enhance arousal.

- **Visual Stimulation:** Engage in eye contact or suggestive glances with your partner. The act of being seen can be incredibly arousing, turning the public setting into a playground of desire.

Incorporating Playful Elements

Adding playful elements can enhance the experience and create a sense of adventure:

- **Role Play:** Consider incorporating role-play scenarios that fit the public setting. For example, pretending to be strangers meeting for the first time can add an exciting layer of anonymity and intrigue.

- **Teasing:** Engage in teasing behaviors that build anticipation. This could involve subtle touches, playful banter, or even light bondage elements that can be easily concealed.

- **Games:** Introduce playful challenges or dares related to the public setting. For instance, taking turns to initiate intimate touches while navigating the space can create a thrilling dynamic.

Addressing Potential Problems

While public breeding scenes can be exhilarating, they also come with potential challenges. Consider the following issues and strategies for resolution:

- **Unwanted Attention:** If you attract unwanted attention, have an exit strategy in place. This could involve moving to a more secluded area or pausing the scene until the situation is under control.

- **Legal Considerations:** Be aware of local laws regarding public displays of affection and sexual activity. Researching the legalities of your chosen location can prevent potential legal issues.

- **Emotional Responses:** Public scenes can evoke strong emotions. Be prepared for the possibility of feelings of vulnerability or anxiety. Engage in aftercare practices to ensure emotional well-being post-scene.

Conclusion

Maximizing pleasure in public breeding scenes requires a delicate balance of excitement, safety, and consent. By thoughtfully selecting locations, negotiating boundaries, enhancing sensory experiences, and addressing potential problems, participants can create an exhilarating and fulfilling experience. The thrill of public intimacy can lead to deeper connections and unforgettable memories, encouraging exploration and enjoyment of one's desires in a shared, adventurous context.

Negotiating Boundaries and Privacy in Public Breeding Scenes

Public breeding scenes can evoke a thrilling blend of excitement and vulnerability. The very nature of these encounters necessitates a robust framework for negotiating boundaries and ensuring privacy, as the stakes are heightened in shared spaces. This section will explore the essential components of boundary negotiation and privacy considerations, providing practical strategies for individuals and groups engaging in public breeding.

Understanding Boundaries in Public Spaces

Boundaries are the invisible lines that define personal comfort zones and dictate acceptable behavior in any interaction. In the context of public breeding scenes, boundaries become even more critical due to the presence of onlookers and the potential for unsolicited attention.

Types of Boundaries Boundaries can be categorized into several types:

- **Physical Boundaries:** These involve personal space and physical contact limits. It is crucial to establish how close others can get and what forms of touch are acceptable.

- **Emotional Boundaries:** Participants must agree on the emotional engagement allowed during the scene. This includes discussing what feelings may arise and how they will be handled.

- **Social Boundaries:** These boundaries pertain to the interaction with the environment and bystanders. Participants should decide how they will respond to external reactions and what behaviors are acceptable in public.

Communicating Boundaries Effectively

Effective communication is the cornerstone of boundary negotiation. It ensures that all participants are on the same page and that their limits are respected.

Establishing Pre-Scene Agreements Before engaging in public breeding, it is essential to have a pre-scene discussion that covers:

- Individual comfort levels with public displays of affection (PDA).

- Specific actions that are off-limits (e.g., certain sexual acts, nudity).

- The use of safe words or signals that can be employed if someone feels uncomfortable.

Utilizing Safe Words Safe words serve as a crucial tool for maintaining safety and consent. In public settings, it can be beneficial to establish a discreet safe word or gesture that can be used to halt the scene without drawing attention. For example, a simple hand signal or a phrase that sounds innocuous can be employed to communicate discomfort.

Privacy Considerations

Privacy in public breeding scenes is multifaceted, involving both physical privacy and the management of personal information.

Location Selection Choosing the right location is paramount. Ideal spots should balance visibility with discretion. For instance, secluded areas in parks or private event spaces can offer the thrill of being in public while maintaining a degree of privacy.

Managing Onlookers It is vital to have a plan for managing potential onlookers. This might include:

- Establishing a perimeter: Designating a physical space that is off-limits to bystanders can help create a sense of privacy.

- Engaging with bystanders: If approached, having a pre-agreed method of interacting with curious onlookers can mitigate discomfort. This could range from friendly banter to politely declining engagement.

Legal and Ethical Considerations

Engaging in public breeding scenes raises legal and ethical questions that must be navigated carefully.

Understanding Local Laws Before participating in public breeding, it is imperative to familiarize oneself with local laws regarding public indecency and sexual conduct. Different jurisdictions have varying definitions of what constitutes acceptable behavior in public spaces.

Ethical Engagement Ethically, it is crucial to consider the comfort and consent of not just participants but also potential witnesses. This may involve:

- Avoiding locations where individuals may inadvertently witness the scene, such as family-oriented areas.

- Being respectful of the environment and ensuring that the scene does not disrupt the public space or infringe on others' rights.

Conclusion

Negotiating boundaries and privacy in public breeding scenes is a complex but rewarding endeavor. By establishing clear communication, selecting appropriate locations, and remaining mindful of legal and ethical considerations, participants can create a thrilling and consensual experience. The key lies in mutual respect and understanding, ensuring that all involved can enjoy the excitement of public breeding while feeling safe and secure.

Total Comfort = Effective Communication+Respect for Boundaries+Privacy Management
(23)

Building Community and Connection through Public Breeding

Public breeding scenes can serve as a unique avenue for fostering community and connection among individuals who share similar desires and fantasies. Engaging in these experiences in a consensual and respectful environment allows participants to explore their sexuality while simultaneously creating bonds with like-minded individuals. This section delves into the theories of community building, the potential challenges faced in public breeding settings, and practical examples of how to cultivate a supportive atmosphere.

Theoretical Framework

The concept of community in the context of public breeding can be analyzed through various sociological theories, such as *Social Identity Theory* (Tajfel & Turner, 1979). This theory posits that individuals derive a sense of identity and self-esteem from their membership in social groups. In public breeding scenarios, individuals may identify with a community that embraces alternative sexual practices, leading to increased self-acceptance and a sense of belonging.

Furthermore, *Communal Reinforcement Theory* suggests that shared experiences can enhance group cohesion. When participants engage in public breeding, they create a collective memory that strengthens their connection to one another. This shared experience can foster trust, openness, and a deeper understanding of each other's desires and boundaries.

Challenges in Public Breeding

While public breeding can be a fulfilling experience, it is not without its challenges. Some potential issues include:

- **Legal and Ethical Concerns:** Engaging in sexual activities in public spaces may lead to legal repercussions. It is crucial to be aware of local laws and regulations regarding public sexual behavior to avoid legal complications.

- **Privacy and Safety:** Public settings can pose risks to personal safety and privacy. Participants must be vigilant about their surroundings and ensure that consent is maintained throughout the experience.

- **Social Stigma:** Individuals may face judgment or stigma from those who do not understand or accept alternative sexual practices. Building a supportive community can help counteract this negativity and provide a safe space for expression.

Creating a Supportive Environment

To build a community around public breeding, it is essential to create a supportive and inclusive environment. Here are some strategies to achieve this:

1. **Establish Clear Guidelines:** Before engaging in public breeding, participants should agree on clear guidelines and boundaries. This includes discussing what behaviors are acceptable, establishing safe words, and ensuring that all parties are comfortable with the chosen setting.

2. **Facilitate Open Communication:** Encourage participants to share their desires, limits, and concerns openly. This can be facilitated through pre-scene discussions, group meetings, or online forums where individuals can express their thoughts without fear of judgment.

3. **Host Community Events:** Organizing events specifically for public breeding can help bring individuals together. These gatherings can range from casual meet-ups to more structured play parties, providing a platform for participants to connect and share experiences.

4. **Utilize Technology:** Online platforms and social media can serve as valuable tools for building community. Creating dedicated groups or forums allows individuals to connect, share advice, and plan public breeding events while maintaining a level of anonymity.

5. **Encourage Inclusivity:** Ensure that your community welcomes individuals of all backgrounds, orientations, and experiences. This inclusivity fosters a sense of belonging and encourages diverse perspectives within the group.

Examples of Community Building

To illustrate the process of building community through public breeding, consider the following examples:

- **Public Play Parties:** Organizing themed play parties in private venues can create a safe space for individuals to explore their desires openly. These events can include workshops on consent and communication, enhancing participants' understanding of each other's needs.

- **Social Media Campaigns:** Launching a campaign to celebrate public breeding can raise awareness and encourage discussions around the topic. This can include sharing personal stories, educational content, and resources for those interested in exploring public breeding.

- **Collaborative Workshops:** Hosting workshops that focus on skills relevant to public breeding—such as negotiation techniques, safety practices, and emotional aftercare—can empower participants and strengthen community ties.

Conclusion

Building community and connection through public breeding is a multifaceted endeavor that requires careful consideration of individual needs, safety, and consent. By fostering open communication, establishing guidelines, and creating inclusive environments, participants can cultivate a supportive community that enhances their public breeding experiences. Embracing the shared journey of exploration and connection can lead to profound personal growth and a deeper understanding of one's desires.

References:
Tajfel, H., & Turner, J. C. (1979). An Integrative Theory of Intergroup Conflict. In *The Social Psychology of Intergroup Relations* (pp. 33-47). Monterey, CA: Brooks/Cole.

Mental and Emotional Well-being in Breeding Scenes

Processing and Aftercare

Debriefing and Communicating Post-Scene

After an intense breeding scene, the importance of debriefing cannot be overstated. This process serves as a bridge between the heightened emotions experienced during the scene and the return to everyday life. It is an opportunity to reflect on the experience, communicate feelings, and ensure that all participants feel safe and respected.

The Importance of Debriefing

Debriefing is a crucial component of any intimate encounter, particularly in breeding scenes where emotional and physical boundaries are often tested. The significance of this process can be outlined in several key areas:

- **Emotional Processing:** Engaging in a breeding scene can elicit a wide range of emotions, from pleasure to vulnerability. Debriefing allows participants to process these feelings in a supportive environment.

- **Reinforcing Consent:** Open communication post-scene helps to reaffirm the consent given before and during the encounter. Discussing what was enjoyable and what may have crossed boundaries is essential for future interactions.

- **Building Trust:** Sharing experiences fosters a deeper connection and trust between partners. This trust is vital for maintaining a healthy and fulfilling breeding lifestyle.

- **Identifying Areas for Improvement:** Debriefing provides a platform to discuss what worked well and what could be improved in future scenes, enhancing the overall experience.

Effective Debriefing Techniques

To facilitate a productive debriefing session, consider the following techniques:

1. **Set Aside Time:** Schedule a dedicated time for debriefing after the scene. This ensures that all participants are mentally prepared to engage in this important conversation.

2. **Create a Safe Space:** Choose a comfortable environment where participants feel safe to express their thoughts and feelings without fear of judgment.

3. **Use Open-Ended Questions:** Encourage dialogue by asking open-ended questions such as:
   - "What was your favorite part of the scene?"
   - "Did anything surprise you during our encounter?"
   - "Is there anything you would like to explore further in the future?"

4. **Practice Active Listening:** Ensure that each participant feels heard. Validate their feelings and experiences, and refrain from interrupting while they share.

5. **Discuss Boundaries:** Revisit the boundaries established prior to the scene. Discuss any moments where those boundaries may have been tested and how they were navigated.

Addressing Emotional Challenges

It is not uncommon for participants to experience emotional challenges after a breeding scene. These may include feelings of guilt, shame, or even confusion about the experience. Addressing these challenges is crucial for emotional well-being.

- **Normalize Feelings:** Remind participants that it is normal to have complex feelings after an intense experience. Encourage them to express any discomfort they may be experiencing.

- **Explore Triggers:** Help identify any specific triggers that may have arisen during the scene. Understanding these triggers can aid in managing them in future encounters.

- **Seek Support:** If emotional challenges persist, suggest seeking support from a therapist or counselor who specializes in alternative lifestyles. Professional guidance can provide valuable tools for navigating these feelings.

Examples of Post-Scene Communication

Here are a few examples of how to initiate post-scene communication:

"I really enjoyed how you took control during the scene. It made me feel deeply connected to you. How did you feel about it?"

"I loved the intensity of our breeding scene, but I felt a bit overwhelmed at one point. Can we talk about that?"

"I think we explored some exciting boundaries today. What are your thoughts on trying something similar next time?"

Conclusion

In conclusion, debriefing and communicating post-scene is an essential practice for anyone engaging in breeding scenes. By fostering open dialogue, addressing emotional challenges, and reinforcing consent, participants can enhance their experiences and build deeper connections. Remember, the journey does not end with the scene; it continues through the conversations that follow. Embrace the opportunity to reflect, learn, and grow together in your erotic lifestyle.

Addressing Any Emotional Challenges

Engaging in breeding scenes can evoke a range of emotions, both during and after the experience. It is crucial to address these emotional challenges to foster a healthy and fulfilling breeding lifestyle. This section explores common emotional responses, the underlying theories, and practical strategies for managing these feelings.

Understanding Emotional Responses

Breeding scenes often involve intense vulnerability and intimacy, which can lead to various emotional challenges, including:

- **Post-Scene Blues:** After an intense experience, individuals may feel a sense of emptiness or sadness, often referred to as "post-scene blues." This phenomenon can occur due to the abrupt transition from heightened arousal to a more mundane state.

- **Anxiety and Insecurity:** Participants may experience anxiety about their performance, their partner's satisfaction, or the implications of their desires. This anxiety can stem from societal stigma surrounding breeding and alternative lifestyles.

- **Jealousy and Comparison:** In group settings, feelings of jealousy may arise, particularly if one partner receives more attention or affection. This can lead to feelings of inadequacy or competition among participants.

- **Emotional Vulnerability:** The intimate nature of breeding scenes may bring unresolved emotional issues to the surface, leading to feelings of fear, shame, or inadequacy.

Theoretical Framework

To better understand these emotional challenges, we can draw on several psychological theories:

- **Attachment Theory:** This theory posits that our early relationships with caregivers shape our emotional responses in adult relationships. Individuals with insecure attachment styles may struggle more with feelings of anxiety or jealousy in breeding scenarios.

- **Cognitive Behavioral Theory (CBT):** CBT suggests that our thoughts influence our emotions and behaviors. Negative thought patterns, such as catastrophizing or all-or-nothing thinking, can exacerbate emotional challenges. For example, a participant may think, "If I don't perform perfectly, I'm a failure," leading to increased anxiety.

- **Emotional Regulation Theory:** This theory emphasizes the importance of managing and responding to emotional experiences. Effective emotional regulation strategies can mitigate negative feelings and enhance overall well-being.

Practical Strategies for Addressing Emotional Challenges

To navigate emotional challenges effectively, consider implementing the following strategies:

1. **Open Communication:** Establish a debriefing process after each breeding scene. Encourage all participants to share their feelings, concerns, and experiences. Use open-ended questions to facilitate dialogue, such as:

"How did you feel during the scene?"

This practice fosters emotional intimacy and allows for the expression of any lingering feelings.

2. **Practice Self-Compassion:** Encourage participants to treat themselves with kindness and understanding. Remind them that experiencing emotional challenges is a normal part of engaging in intimate activities. A self-compassionate mantra might be:

"It's okay to feel this way; I am doing my best."

3. **Journaling:** Keeping a journal can be an effective way to process emotions. Participants can write about their experiences, feelings, and any challenges they faced. This practice can help clarify thoughts and promote emotional healing.

4. **Seek Professional Support:** If emotional challenges persist or become overwhelming, consider seeking support from a therapist specializing in alternative lifestyles or sexual health. Professional guidance can provide valuable tools for managing emotions and enhancing overall well-being.

5. **Engage in Aftercare:** Aftercare is crucial in addressing emotional challenges. It involves providing physical and emotional support to one another after a breeding scene. This can include cuddling, discussing the experience, or simply being present for each other. Aftercare helps reinforce trust and connection, easing emotional turbulence.

Conclusion

Addressing emotional challenges in breeding scenes is essential for creating a safe and fulfilling experience. By understanding the emotional landscape and implementing effective strategies, participants can navigate their feelings with grace and resilience. Remember that emotional challenges are not a sign of weakness; they are a natural part of exploring one's desires and fostering deep connections in the breeding lifestyle.

Seeking Professional Support if Needed

In the journey of exploring breeding scenes, it is crucial to acknowledge that emotional and psychological well-being is paramount. Engaging in such intimate and often intense experiences can stir a multitude of feelings, from excitement and pleasure to anxiety and vulnerability. Therefore, seeking professional support can be a vital step in ensuring a healthy and fulfilling breeding lifestyle.

Understanding the Need for Support

It is not uncommon for individuals to experience emotional challenges after participating in breeding scenes. These challenges may include feelings of guilt, confusion, or even regret. According to the *American Psychological Association*, engaging in sexual practices that challenge societal norms can lead to psychological stress, especially if those practices are not fully understood or accepted by oneself or one's community.

Theories such as *Attachment Theory* suggest that our early relationships shape our emotional responses and behaviors in adult relationships. This framework can help individuals understand their feelings about breeding and intimacy. For instance, someone with an anxious attachment style may struggle with feelings of insecurity or fear of abandonment after a breeding scene, making professional support beneficial.

When to Seek Help

Recognizing when to seek professional support is essential. Signs that you may benefit from speaking to a professional include:

- Persistent feelings of anxiety or depression related to your sexual experiences.

- Difficulty processing emotions or experiences after engaging in breeding scenes.

- Conflicts arising in relationships due to differing views on breeding practices.

- An overwhelming sense of shame or guilt associated with your desires.

- Feeling isolated or misunderstood in your community regarding your interests.

Types of Professionals to Consider

When seeking support, various professionals can provide assistance:

- **Therapists and Counselors:** Look for those who specialize in sexual health, alternative lifestyles, or kink-aware therapy. They can help you navigate your feelings and provide coping strategies.

- **Sex Educators and Coaches:** These professionals can offer insights into healthy sexual practices and help you understand your desires better, fostering a positive relationship with your sexuality.

- **Medical Experts:** If you have health concerns related to your sexual practices, consulting a healthcare provider specializing in sexual health is crucial. They can provide guidance on safe practices and address any physical concerns.

Approaching the Conversation

When approaching a professional, consider the following steps to ensure a productive dialogue:

- **Be Honest and Open:** Share your experiences, feelings, and concerns without fear of judgment. A good professional will create a safe space for you to express yourself.

- **Set Goals for Therapy:** Identify what you hope to achieve from your sessions. This could range from processing specific experiences to developing healthier coping mechanisms.

- **Ask Questions:** Inquire about their experience with alternative lifestyles and breeding practices. It is essential to work with someone who understands your context.

Examples of Scenarios Requiring Support

Consider the following scenarios that illustrate when seeking professional support may be particularly beneficial:

- **Post-Scene Reflection:** After a particularly intense breeding scene, an individual may feel a mix of exhilaration and dread. A therapist can help unpack these feelings, exploring the underlying reasons for such emotional responses.

- **Relationship Dynamics:** A couple engaged in breeding practices may find that their differing comfort levels lead to tension. A sex educator can facilitate discussions about boundaries and desires, fostering better communication.

- **Coping with Social Stigma:** An individual may feel isolated due to societal stigma surrounding breeding scenes. A support group led by a trained professional can provide a sense of community and understanding, helping individuals navigate their feelings of alienation.

Conclusion

Seeking professional support is not a sign of weakness; rather, it is a proactive step toward emotional health and well-being. Engaging in breeding scenes can be a rewarding experience, but it is essential to ensure that your mental and emotional needs are met. By recognizing the importance of professional guidance, you can navigate your breeding lifestyle with confidence and clarity, ultimately enhancing your overall experience.

Self-Care Practices for Emotional Wellness in Breeding

In the realm of breeding scenes, where the lines of pleasure and emotional connection intertwine, self-care becomes an essential practice for maintaining emotional wellness. Engaging in breeding dynamics can evoke a spectrum of emotions, from euphoria and intimacy to vulnerability and anxiety. Therefore, developing a self-care routine tailored to the unique experiences of breeding is crucial for sustaining mental health and fostering a positive environment for all participants.

Understanding Emotional Responses

Breeding scenes often elicit profound emotional responses. The thrill of surrendering to desire can be exhilarating, yet it may also trigger feelings of insecurity or fear. Understanding the duality of these emotions is vital. According to the *Cognitive-Behavioral Theory*, our thoughts influence our feelings and behaviors. Thus, acknowledging and reframing negative thoughts can mitigate emotional distress. For example, if one feels anxious about their performance, they might remind themselves that the experience is about mutual pleasure and connection, not perfection.

Practicing Mindfulness and Grounding Techniques

Mindfulness practices can significantly enhance emotional wellness in breeding contexts. Engaging in mindfulness involves being present in the moment and accepting one's feelings without judgment. Techniques such as deep breathing, meditation, or body scanning can help individuals center themselves before and after scenes. For instance, before entering a breeding scene, participants can practice a simple breathing exercise:

Inhale deeply through the nose for 4 seconds, hold for 4 seconds, and exhale through the m
(24)

This technique not only calms the mind but also prepares the body for the sensory experiences ahead.

Grounding techniques, such as focusing on physical sensations (the feel of the sheets, the warmth of a partner's skin), can help individuals remain anchored during intense emotional moments. This practice can prevent feelings of overwhelm and promote a sense of safety.

Establishing a Post-Scene Routine

Aftercare is an integral aspect of breeding scenes that directly contributes to emotional wellness. Aftercare involves the practices and rituals that follow a scene, ensuring that all participants feel cared for and connected. This can include cuddling, discussing the experience, and engaging in comforting activities such as sharing a warm drink or taking a bath together.

Creating a structured post-scene routine can help individuals process their emotions. For example, participants might take turns sharing their feelings about the scene, discussing what they enjoyed, and addressing any discomfort. This open dialogue fosters trust and reinforces emotional bonds.

Engaging in Reflective Practices

Reflective practices are vital for understanding one's emotional landscape in breeding dynamics. Journaling can be a powerful tool for processing feelings and experiences. Participants can write about their thoughts before and after scenes, exploring what aspects brought them joy or discomfort. This practice not only aids in emotional processing but also helps identify patterns in one's reactions.

Additionally, engaging in discussions with trusted partners or friends can provide valuable insights. Sharing experiences and feelings can normalize emotional responses and foster a sense of community.

Utilizing Creative Outlets for Expression

Creative expression can serve as a therapeutic outlet for processing emotions related to breeding. Activities such as drawing, painting, or writing erotic fiction can help individuals explore their desires and feelings in a safe space. For instance, writing a short story inspired by a breeding scene can allow one to delve deeper into their fantasies and emotional responses, promoting self-discovery and acceptance.

Seeking Professional Support

In some cases, emotional challenges may require professional guidance. Therapists specializing in alternative lifestyles can provide valuable support and strategies for managing complex emotions arising from breeding scenes. Engaging in therapy can help individuals navigate feelings of shame, anxiety, or insecurity, fostering a healthier relationship with their sexuality.

Conclusion

Self-care practices are not merely an afterthought but a vital component of emotional wellness in breeding scenes. By incorporating mindfulness, establishing aftercare routines, engaging in reflective practices, utilizing creative outlets, and seeking professional support when necessary, individuals can enhance their emotional resilience and enrich their breeding experiences. Ultimately, prioritizing emotional wellness not only benefits the individual but also cultivates deeper connections and satisfaction within the breeding community.

Techniques for Emotional Connection and Bonding in Breeding

Creating emotional connections during breeding scenes is essential for fostering intimacy and trust between partners. This section explores various techniques that can enhance emotional bonding, ensuring that the experience is fulfilling on both physical and emotional levels.

Understanding Emotional Connection

Emotional connection can be defined as the sense of closeness and understanding that partners share. According to attachment theory, individuals develop patterns

PROCESSING AND AFTERCARE 151

of attachment based on their early relationships, which can influence their adult relationships. Breeding scenes often evoke deep emotional responses, making it crucial to establish a secure emotional environment.

Techniques for Enhancing Emotional Bonding

1. **Establishing Intimacy through Eye Contact:** Eye contact can significantly enhance emotional connection. During breeding, maintaining eye contact can create a powerful bond, allowing partners to feel seen and understood. Research shows that prolonged eye contact can increase feelings of attraction and intimacy [?].

2. **Engaging in Deep Conversations:** Before and after breeding scenes, engaging in meaningful conversations can help partners understand each other's desires and boundaries. Discussing fantasies, fears, and experiences can create a safe space where both partners feel valued. This dialogue can include questions such as:

    - What does breeding mean to you?
    - How do you feel during and after a breeding scene?
    - What are your boundaries and desires in this context?

3. **Practicing Vulnerability:** Sharing personal stories and vulnerabilities can deepen emotional intimacy. This practice allows partners to connect on a more profound level, fostering trust. For instance, discussing past experiences related to breeding or emotional responses can help create a supportive environment.

4. **Incorporating Aftercare:** Aftercare is crucial in any BDSM or breeding scene, as it provides an opportunity for partners to reconnect emotionally after the intensity of the experience. Aftercare can involve cuddling, discussing the scene, or simply being present with each other. According to a study by [?], aftercare can significantly impact emotional well-being post-scene.

5. **Utilizing Sensory Experiences:** Engaging the senses can enhance emotional bonding. Consider incorporating elements such as scented candles, soft music, or textured fabrics to create a sensory-rich environment. These elements can evoke feelings of comfort and safety, allowing partners to relax and connect emotionally.

6. **Creating Rituals:** Establishing rituals before or after breeding scenes can enhance emotional connections. Rituals may include specific warm-up activities, shared affirmations, or post-scene reflections. These practices can create a sense of continuity and deepen the emotional bond over time.

7. **Exploring Shared Fantasies:** Discussing and exploring shared fantasies can enhance emotional intimacy. When partners engage in fantasies together, it creates a unique bond based on mutual trust and understanding. This exploration can include roleplay scenarios that resonate with both partners, deepening their emotional connection.

Addressing Potential Challenges

While fostering emotional connections is vital, challenges may arise. Partners may experience feelings of insecurity, jealousy, or vulnerability during breeding scenes. Here are some strategies to address these challenges:

- **Open Communication:** Encourage partners to express their feelings openly. This communication can help identify any insecurities or concerns that may arise during breeding.

- **Setting Clear Boundaries:** Establishing and respecting boundaries can prevent misunderstandings and ensure that both partners feel safe and secure. Use negotiation techniques discussed in Section 3.1 to clarify boundaries.

- **Regular Check-ins:** Aftercare should include regular emotional check-ins to discuss feelings and experiences. This practice can help partners navigate any emotional challenges that arise.

Conclusion

Emotional connection and bonding are integral to enhancing the breeding experience. By incorporating techniques such as establishing intimacy through eye contact, engaging in deep conversations, practicing vulnerability, and utilizing sensory experiences, partners can create a fulfilling emotional environment. Addressing potential challenges through open communication and regular check-ins can further strengthen these connections, leading to a more satisfying and intimate breeding experience.

Conclusion

Embracing the Breeding Lifestyle

Reflecting on Your Journey

As you stand at the crossroads of your erotic lifestyle, reflecting on your journey is not merely an exercise in nostalgia; it is a vital component of growth and self-discovery. The act of reflection allows you to examine the experiences that have shaped your desires, the boundaries you have explored, and the connections you have forged through breeding scenes. This section will delve into the importance of reflection, the theories that underpin it, and practical approaches to guide you in this introspective process.

The Importance of Reflection

Reflection serves multiple purposes in your breeding lifestyle. Firstly, it fosters self-awareness, enabling you to understand your motivations, desires, and limits. According to Kolb's Experiential Learning Theory, learning is a process whereby knowledge is created through the transformation of experience. This theory posits that reflection is a critical stage in the learning cycle, allowing individuals to analyze their experiences and derive meaningful insights.

Learning Cycle = Concrete Experience → Reflective Observation → Abstract Conceptua
(25)

By engaging in reflective observation, you can assess your experiences in breeding scenes, considering what worked well and what did not. This process not only enhances your understanding of your erotic preferences but also encourages personal growth.

Identifying Key Experiences

To facilitate reflection, identify key experiences in your breeding journey. These may include:

- **First Breeding Scene:** Recall your initial foray into breeding. What emotions did you experience? How did it shape your understanding of pleasure and intimacy?

- **Memorable Connections:** Reflect on significant encounters with partners. What made these connections special? How did they enhance your experience of breeding?

- **Challenges Faced:** Consider any obstacles you encountered, such as miscommunication or emotional discomfort. What lessons did these challenges teach you about consent and boundaries?

As you reflect on these experiences, consider journaling your thoughts. Writing can be a cathartic process, helping to clarify your feelings and track your growth over time.

Theoretical Frameworks for Reflection

In addition to Kolb's theory, other psychological frameworks can enrich your reflective practice. The *Gibbs Reflective Cycle* is particularly useful for structuring your reflections. This model consists of six stages:

1. **Description:** What happened during your breeding scenes?

2. **Feelings:** What were your emotional responses?

3. **Evaluation:** What was good and bad about the experience?

4. **Analysis:** What sense can you make of the situation?

5. **Conclusion:** What else could you have done?

6. **Action Plan:** If faced with a similar situation again, what would you do?

Applying Gibbs' cycle to your breeding experiences can help you gain deeper insights and develop actionable strategies for future encounters.

Examples of Reflective Practice

To illustrate the reflective process, consider the following hypothetical scenarios:

> **Example**
>
> Scenario 1: A Positive Experience
> You participated in a breeding scene that left you feeling euphoric and deeply connected to your partner. In your reflection, you might describe the heightened sense of intimacy and the trust that was established. You could evaluate the factors that contributed to this experience, such as effective communication and a well-prepared environment. Your action plan may involve replicating these elements in future scenes.

> **Example**
>
> Scenario 2: A Challenging Experience
> During a group breeding scene, you felt overwhelmed by the dynamics at play. Reflecting on this experience, you might identify feelings of anxiety and discomfort. Evaluating the situation could reveal that boundaries were not clearly established. Your conclusion might emphasize the importance of pre-scene negotiations, leading to an action plan focused on improving communication in future group settings.

Integrating Reflection into Your Lifestyle

To make reflection a regular part of your breeding lifestyle, consider incorporating the following practices:

- **Regular Journaling:** Set aside time each week to document your thoughts and feelings about your experiences.

- **Partner Discussions:** Engage in open conversations with your partners about your experiences, desires, and boundaries. This can deepen your connection and foster mutual understanding.

- **Workshops and Support Groups:** Participate in events that focus on reflection and personal growth within the erotic community. Sharing experiences with like-minded individuals can provide new perspectives and insights.

Conclusion

Reflecting on your journey in the breeding lifestyle is not just about looking back; it is about using your past experiences to inform your future. By understanding your desires, learning from challenges, and celebrating successes, you can continue to evolve in your erotic journey. Embrace the process of reflection as a tool for empowerment, allowing you to navigate the complexities of your breeding lifestyle with confidence and clarity.

As you conclude this section, remember that reflection is an ongoing process. Each experience, whether pleasurable or challenging, contributes to your understanding of yourself and your desires. Embrace this journey of self-discovery, and let it guide you towards deeper connections and more fulfilling experiences in your breeding lifestyle.

Continuing to Explore and Experiment

In the realm of breeding scenes, the journey of exploration and experimentation is an essential aspect of deepening your understanding and enhancing your pleasure. As you continue to navigate your desires, it is crucial to approach this exploration with an open mind and a willingness to adapt. The following sections will delve into various strategies for ongoing experimentation, emphasizing the importance of creativity, communication, and safety.

Embracing New Experiences

One of the most significant aspects of the breeding lifestyle is the opportunity to embrace new experiences. This can involve trying out different roles, settings, or techniques. For example, if you have primarily engaged in private breeding scenes, consider exploring the thrill of public settings. The excitement of being in a semi-public space can heighten arousal and deepen the connection between partners.

Role Exploration

Role exploration can also add depth to your breeding experiences. Experimenting with different dynamics can lead to heightened pleasure and satisfaction. For instance, if you typically assume a submissive role, consider switching roles with your partner to experience the power dynamics from a different perspective. This shift can provide valuable insights into your desires and boundaries.

Incorporating New Techniques

Incorporating new techniques into your breeding scenes can enhance pleasure and satisfaction. For example, consider exploring the use of toys or accessories that you haven't previously utilized. This could range from simple items like blindfolds to more intricate devices designed for prostate stimulation. Each new tool can introduce different sensations, allowing for a richer breeding experience.

Communicating Desires and Boundaries

As you explore and experiment, communication remains paramount. Engaging in open and honest discussions with your partner about your desires and boundaries is crucial for a fulfilling experience. Establishing a safe word or signal can provide an additional layer of security, allowing both partners to express discomfort or the need to pause without fear of judgment.

Theoretical Frameworks for Exploration

To further understand the dynamics of exploration, consider the theoretical framework of *sexual fluidity*. This concept suggests that sexual attraction and desire can change over time and in different contexts. By recognizing that your preferences may evolve, you can approach your breeding lifestyle with flexibility and openness.

Balancing Safety and Adventure

While experimentation is vital, it is equally important to maintain a balance between safety and adventure. Before venturing into new territories, ensure that both partners are comfortable with the proposed activities. Discuss health and safety concerns, and consider establishing a checklist of practices that prioritize well-being.

Example of a Breeding Scene Experimentation

Consider a scenario where a couple has primarily engaged in traditional breeding scenes. To explore new dimensions, they decide to incorporate roleplay into their next encounter. One partner takes on the role of a dominant figure, while the other embodies a submissive persona. They set the scene with props, such as a collar and leash, to enhance the experience.

During this encounter, they communicate openly about their feelings and reactions, allowing for adjustments as needed. This experimentation not only deepens their connection but also fosters trust and intimacy.

Reflecting on Experiences

After each exploration, take the time to reflect on the experience. What did you enjoy? What could be improved? This reflection process is crucial for growth and understanding in your breeding journey. Consider keeping a journal to document your thoughts and feelings, creating a personal archive of your evolving desires and experiences.

Continuing Education

Lastly, consider engaging in continuous education regarding your breeding lifestyle. Attend workshops, read literature, and participate in discussions within your community. Staying informed will empower you to make educated choices about your exploration and keep your experiences fresh and exciting.

In conclusion, continuing to explore and experiment within the breeding lifestyle is essential for personal growth and satisfaction. By embracing new experiences, communicating openly, and maintaining a balance between safety and adventure, you can deepen your connection with yourself and your partners. Remember, the journey is ongoing, and each new experience can lead to greater understanding and pleasure.

Staying Safe and Satisfied

In the realm of erotic exploration, particularly within breeding scenes, the dual pillars of safety and satisfaction are paramount. Engaging in such intimate activities requires a conscious commitment to both physical and emotional well-being. This section delves into strategies for ensuring that your experiences are not only fulfilling but also secure.

Understanding Safety in Breeding Scenes

Safety in breeding scenes encompasses a variety of aspects, including physical health, emotional readiness, and the establishment of a supportive environment. The foundation of safety lies in the principles of consent, communication, and preparation.

Physical Health Considerations Before embarking on breeding scenes, it is crucial to address health concerns. Regular sexual health check-ups are essential for all participants. This includes testing for sexually transmitted infections (STIs) and discussing birth control options. The use of condoms can significantly reduce the risk of STIs and unintended pregnancies, while also enhancing the safety of the experience.

$$\text{Safety Index} = \frac{\text{Health Precautions}}{\text{Risk Factors}}$$

Where:

- **Health Precautions** includes the use of protection, regular health screenings, and open discussions about sexual health.

- **Risk Factors** encompasses the number of partners, lack of communication, and absence of safety protocols.

Emotional Safety and Readiness

The emotional landscape of breeding scenes can be complex. Participants should engage in self-reflection to assess their emotional readiness. Questions to consider include:

- Am I comfortable with the concept of breeding?

- What are my boundaries regarding emotional attachment and intimacy?

- How do I feel about the potential consequences of breeding scenarios?

Communicating Needs and Boundaries Effective communication is the cornerstone of both safety and satisfaction. Prior to engaging in breeding activities, it is essential to have open discussions with partners about desires, boundaries, and safe words. Establishing a safe word or signal can provide a means to pause or stop the scene if discomfort arises.

$$\text{Communication Quality} = \frac{\text{Clarity} + \text{Openness}}{\text{Misunderstandings}}$$

Creating a Supportive Environment

The environment in which breeding scenes take place can significantly influence the overall experience. A supportive and comfortable setting can enhance feelings of safety and satisfaction. Consider the following elements:

- **Privacy:** Ensure that the space is private and free from interruptions.

- **Comfort:** Utilize soft furnishings, ambient lighting, and soothing music to create a relaxing atmosphere.

- **Accessibility:** Make sure that all participants can easily access necessary items, such as water, protection, and aftercare supplies.

Aftercare: The Key to Satisfaction

Aftercare is an essential component of any breeding scene. It involves the emotional and physical support provided to partners after intense activities. The importance of aftercare cannot be overstated; it helps to reinforce trust, intimacy, and satisfaction.

Techniques for Effective Aftercare

- **Debriefing:** Engage in a conversation about the experience, discussing what was enjoyable and any discomforts that arose.

- **Physical Comfort:** Provide cuddling, gentle touch, or a warm drink to help partners relax and feel cared for.

- **Emotional Support:** Be attentive to each other's emotional needs, validating feelings and offering reassurance.

Addressing Common Problems

Even with the best preparations, problems may arise during breeding scenes. Common issues include miscommunication, emotional distress, or unexpected physical reactions. It is vital to approach these situations with patience and understanding.

Examples of Issues and Solutions

- **Miscommunication:** If a partner expresses discomfort, pause the scene immediately. Revisit the discussion of boundaries and ensure everyone feels heard.

- **Emotional Distress:** If a participant experiences unexpected feelings of anxiety or sadness, provide space for them to express their emotions. Engage in aftercare practices to help them process these feelings.

- **Physical Reactions:** If a participant experiences pain or discomfort, prioritize their well-being by stopping the activity and assessing the situation.

Conclusion: The Balance of Safety and Satisfaction

In conclusion, staying safe and satisfied in breeding scenes requires a proactive approach to health, communication, and emotional well-being. By prioritizing these elements, participants can create enriching experiences that foster deep connections and mutual pleasure. Embrace the journey of exploration with mindfulness, ensuring that safety and satisfaction are always at the forefront of your breeding lifestyle.

$$\text{Overall Satisfaction} = \frac{\text{Physical Safety} + \text{Emotional Security} + \text{Effective Communication}}{\text{Potential Risks}}$$

Where:

- **Physical Safety** pertains to health precautions and protection measures.

- **Emotional Security** relates to the comfort and readiness of participants.

- **Effective Communication** involves clear discussions about desires and boundaries.

- **Potential Risks** includes any factors that could compromise safety or satisfaction.

Looking Forward to Future Breeding Adventures

As you embrace the breeding lifestyle, it is essential to maintain an open mindset towards future adventures. The journey of exploring your desires and fantasies does not end with the experiences you have already had; rather, it evolves and expands with each new encounter. In this section, we will explore how to cultivate a forward-looking attitude, the importance of adaptability, and the potential for growth within your breeding experiences.

Embracing Change and Growth

The breeding lifestyle, much like any other aspect of human sexuality, is not static. It is subject to change, influenced by personal growth, relationship dynamics, and evolving desires. Embracing this fluidity can enhance your experiences and deepen your connections with partners.

$$E = mc^2 \tag{26}$$

This famous equation by Einstein, while primarily related to physics, can metaphorically represent the energy exchange in your breeding adventures. Here, E symbolizes the emotional energy shared between partners, m represents the mutual desires and fantasies, and c denotes the connection that amplifies your experiences. As you engage in breeding scenes, consider how your emotional energy can transform and evolve, creating new dimensions of pleasure and intimacy.

Setting Intentions for Future Experiences

Intentions play a crucial role in shaping your breeding adventures. By setting clear intentions, you can navigate your experiences with purpose and clarity. This could involve exploring new techniques, incorporating different partners, or even experimenting with various environments.

- **Example 1:** If you wish to enhance your connection with a partner, consider planning a breeding scene that focuses on deep emotional intimacy. This could involve extended foreplay, eye contact, and verbal affirmations of desire.

- **Example 2:** If you are interested in expanding your breeding circle, set an intention to attend events or gatherings where you can meet like-minded individuals. Engaging in group dynamics can introduce you to new perspectives and experiences.

EMBRACING THE BREEDING LIFESTYLE

Exploring New Techniques and Dynamics

With each new adventure, there is an opportunity to explore different techniques and dynamics within your breeding scenes. This exploration can be both exciting and rewarding, allowing you to discover what resonates with you and your partners.

$$P = \int_a^b f(x)\, dx \qquad (27)$$

In this equation, P represents the pleasure derived from your experiences, while $f(x)$ signifies the various techniques and dynamics you engage with. The integral from a to b reflects the journey of exploration, where each new technique adds to the overall pleasure.

Consider incorporating elements of roleplay, power dynamics, or sensory experiences into your breeding adventures. For instance, if you have primarily engaged in traditional breeding scenes, you might explore the incorporation of BDSM elements or fantasy scenarios to heighten arousal and excitement.

Building a Supportive Community

As you look forward to future breeding adventures, it is vital to surround yourself with a supportive community. Engaging with others who share similar interests can provide encouragement, inspiration, and a wealth of knowledge.

- **Example 3:** Join online forums or local meetups that focus on breeding and related lifestyles. These platforms can serve as valuable resources for sharing experiences, seeking advice, and discovering new opportunities for connection.

- **Example 4:** Attend workshops or seminars that delve into specific aspects of breeding. These educational experiences can enhance your understanding and skills, preparing you for more fulfilling adventures.

Reflecting on Past Experiences

While looking forward is essential, it is equally important to reflect on your past breeding experiences. Consider what you have learned, what brought you joy, and what challenges you encountered. This reflection can inform your future adventures and help you identify patterns or areas for growth.

$$L = \frac{1}{N} \sum_{i=1}^{N} l_i \qquad (28)$$

In this equation, L represents the overall learning derived from your breeding experiences, N is the number of encounters, and l_i denotes the lessons learned from each individual experience. By analyzing your past, you can cultivate a deeper understanding of your desires and preferences, guiding you toward more fulfilling future encounters.

Continuing the Journey

The journey of breeding is an ongoing exploration of intimacy, pleasure, and connection. As you look forward to future adventures, remain open to the possibilities that lie ahead. Each experience is an opportunity to learn, grow, and deepen your understanding of yourself and your partners.

In conclusion, the breeding lifestyle is a rich tapestry woven from the threads of desire, connection, and exploration. By embracing change, setting intentions, exploring new techniques, building community, and reflecting on past experiences, you can enhance your future breeding adventures. Remember, the journey is as important as the destination, and each step along the way contributes to your overall satisfaction and fulfillment in this erotic lifestyle.

Inspiring Others to Embrace Their Desires and Fantasies

Embracing one's desires and fantasies is a deeply personal journey, yet it can also serve as an inspiration for others. The act of sharing our experiences and insights can create a ripple effect, encouraging those around us to explore their own sexual identities and fantasies without fear or shame. This section will delve into the importance of fostering a supportive environment, the theoretical framework behind sexual liberation, and practical steps to inspire others in their journey of self-discovery.

Theoretical Framework of Sexual Liberation

Sexual liberation is grounded in several key theories that emphasize the importance of self-acceptance and the rejection of societal norms that stigmatize sexual expression. One such theory is the **Sexual Liberation Theory**, which posits that individuals should have the autonomy to explore their sexual desires freely, without the constraints of societal expectations. This theory aligns with the works of influential sex educators and psychologists, such as *Dr. Ruth Westheimer* and *Betty Dodson*, who advocate for sexual self-exploration as a path to empowerment.

Additionally, the **Kinsey Scale**, developed by *Alfred Kinsey*, provides a framework for understanding sexual orientation and desire as a spectrum rather than a binary. This perspective encourages individuals to embrace the full range of their sexual identities, paving the way for a more inclusive understanding of breeding scenes and fantasies. The equation that can be derived from Kinsey's work is:

$$S = \frac{D}{T}$$

Where: - S is the spectrum of sexual orientation, - D represents diverse desires, and - T signifies the time spent exploring these desires.

This equation highlights the importance of both diversity in desire and the time dedicated to understanding those desires.

Identifying Barriers to Acceptance

Before inspiring others, it is crucial to recognize the barriers that often inhibit individuals from embracing their desires. These barriers can include:

- **Societal Stigma:** Cultural norms may label certain fantasies as taboo, leading to feelings of guilt or shame.

- **Fear of Judgment:** Individuals may fear being judged by peers or loved ones, which can stifle their willingness to explore their fantasies.

- **Lack of Knowledge:** A limited understanding of sexual health and wellness can deter individuals from pursuing their desires safely and consensually.

- **Internalized Shame:** Past experiences or teachings may lead to internal conflicts regarding one's sexual identity or desires.

Understanding these barriers is essential for creating a supportive environment where individuals feel safe to express themselves.

Practical Steps to Inspire Others

Here are several practical strategies to inspire others to embrace their desires and fantasies:

1. **Share Personal Stories:** Sharing your own experiences with breeding scenes and fantasies can normalize these discussions and encourage others to open up about their desires. Use storytelling techniques to convey your journey authentically, highlighting both challenges and triumphs.

2. **Create Safe Spaces:** Foster environments where individuals feel comfortable discussing their fantasies without judgment. This could be through workshops, discussion groups, or online forums that focus on sexual health and exploration.

3. **Educate on Sexual Health:** Provide resources and information about safe practices, consent, and the benefits of exploring one's sexuality. This education can empower individuals to make informed decisions about their desires.

4. **Encourage Open Dialogue:** Promote conversations about desires and fantasies in your social circles. Use open-ended questions to guide discussions, allowing individuals to express their thoughts and feelings freely.

5. **Lead by Example:** Demonstrate a positive attitude towards sexual exploration. Your confidence in discussing and embracing your desires can inspire others to do the same.

Examples of Inspiration in Action

Consider the case of a local community group that hosts monthly "Desire Nights," where participants are encouraged to share their fantasies and experiences in a supportive setting. These gatherings not only provide a platform for expression but also foster connections among individuals with similar interests.

Another example is the rise of social media platforms dedicated to sexual health and wellness, where influencers share their journeys and encourage followers to embrace their desires. These platforms serve as powerful tools for normalization and inspiration, reaching a wider audience and promoting acceptance.

Conclusion

Inspiring others to embrace their desires and fantasies is a powerful way to foster a culture of acceptance and exploration. By understanding the theoretical frameworks of sexual liberation, identifying barriers to acceptance, and implementing practical strategies, we can create an environment where individuals feel empowered to explore their sexual identities. As we share our stories and support one another, we contribute to a more open and accepting society, where everyone can confidently embrace their desires and fantasies.

Bibliography

[1] Kinsey, A. C. (1948). *Sexual Behavior in the Human Male*. W.B. Saunders Company.

[2] Dodson, B. (1996). *Sex for One: The Joy of Self-Loving*. HarperCollins.

[3] Westheimer, R. (2003). *Dr. Ruth's Guide to Sex*. Grand Central Publishing.

Resources

Recommended Reading

Books on BDSM and Power Dynamics

In the realm of erotic exploration, understanding the intricacies of BDSM and power dynamics is essential for both personal growth and enhancing the experiences shared with partners. This section highlights key texts that delve into the theory, practice, and ethical considerations surrounding BDSM, providing readers with a robust foundation for their journeys into these thrilling territories.

Foundational Texts

One of the most seminal works in the BDSM community is *The New Topping Book* by Dossie Easton and Janet W. Hardy. This book offers an insightful exploration into the mindset of a Dominant partner, emphasizing the importance of communication, consent, and the psychological aspects of power exchange. The authors argue that effective topping requires a deep understanding of one's partner's needs and boundaries, a theme echoed throughout the BDSM literature.

In contrast, *The New Bottoming Book*, also by Easton and Hardy, provides a comprehensive guide for those who identify as submissive. This text explores the emotional and psychological dimensions of submission, discussing how individuals can navigate their desires while maintaining their sense of self. The authors emphasize the importance of self-awareness and negotiation in BDSM relationships, reinforcing the idea that submission is not about relinquishing control but rather about choosing to give it.

Theoretical Perspectives

For a more academic approach, *The BDSM Phenomenon: A Study of Power Exchange in Sexual Relationships* by Dr. Charley Ferrer offers a sociological perspective on BDSM practices. Ferrer's research highlights the diverse motivations behind engaging in BDSM, including the exploration of power, trust, and intimacy. The book examines how these dynamics can foster deeper connections between partners, challenging societal norms surrounding sexuality and relationships.

Additionally, *Playing Well with Others: Your Field Guide to Discovering, Exploring and Navigating the Kink and BDSM Communities* by Lee Harrington and Mollena Williams offers practical advice for those new to the BDSM scene. This guide addresses the complexities of community dynamics, consent, and safety, providing readers with tools to engage in BDSM responsibly. The authors emphasize the importance of informed consent and ongoing communication, essential components for navigating power dynamics in any BDSM encounter.

Practical Guides

For those looking to incorporate BDSM elements into their relationships, *SM 101: A Realistic Introduction* by Jay Wiseman serves as a practical manual. Wiseman covers a range of topics from the basics of bondage to the psychological aspects of sadomasochism. His straightforward approach demystifies BDSM practices and provides readers with the knowledge needed to engage safely and consensually.

Moreover, *The Art of Sensual Female Dominance: A Guide for Women* by Lady Green offers a unique perspective on female empowerment within BDSM. This book explores the nuances of female dominance, providing techniques and insights for women who wish to embrace their Dominant side. Lady Green discusses the psychological aspects of power dynamics, emphasizing the importance of confidence and communication in establishing authority.

Addressing Common Problems

While exploring BDSM and power dynamics can be exhilarating, it is not without its challenges. Miscommunication, lack of consent, and emotional fallout are potential pitfalls that can arise in these relationships. *The Ethical Slut: A Practical Guide to Polyamory, Open Relationships, and Other Adventures* by Dossie Easton and Janet W. Hardy addresses these issues head-on, offering strategies for maintaining healthy relationships within the context of non-monogamy and

BDSM. The authors advocate for open dialogue and continuous consent, encouraging individuals to voice their needs and concerns.

Furthermore, *BDSM and the Politics of Consent* by Dr. Clarisse Thorn examines the complexities of consent in BDSM practices, particularly in relation to societal norms and legal frameworks. Thorn's work challenges readers to consider the implications of consent beyond the bedroom, exploring how power dynamics play out in broader social contexts. This critical analysis is vital for anyone engaged in BDSM, as it encourages a deeper understanding of the ethical considerations involved.

Conclusion

The literature on BDSM and power dynamics is vast and varied, offering a wealth of knowledge for those interested in exploring these themes. From foundational texts that establish the principles of consent and communication to practical guides that provide strategies for navigating relationships, these books serve as essential resources for anyone looking to deepen their understanding of BDSM. By engaging with these texts, readers can enhance their experiences, foster deeper connections with their partners, and embrace the complexities of their desires in a safe and consensual manner.

Recommended Reading:

- Easton, D., & Hardy, J. W. (2014). *The New Topping Book*. Greenery Press.

- Easton, D., & Hardy, J. W. (2014). *The New Bottoming Book*. Greenery Press.

- Ferrer, C. (2016). *The BDSM Phenomenon: A Study of Power Exchange in Sexual Relationships*. CreateSpace Independent Publishing Platform.

- Harrington, L., & Williams, M. (2015). *Playing Well with Others: Your Field Guide to Discovering, Exploring and Navigating the Kink and BDSM Communities*. Greenery Press.

- Wiseman, J. (1996). *SM 101: A Realistic Introduction*. Greenery Press.

- Green, L. (2008). *The Art of Sensual Female Dominance: A Guide for Women*. Greenery Press.

- Easton, D., & Hardy, J. W. (2017). *The Ethical Slut: A Practical Guide to Polyamory, Open Relationships, and Other Adventures*. Ten Speed Press.

- Thorn, C. (2012). *BDSM and the Politics of Consent*. CreateSpace Independent Publishing Platform.

RESOURCES

Literature on Sexual Health and Wellness

The exploration of sexual health and wellness is an essential component of understanding breeding scenes and the broader erotic lifestyle. This literature encompasses a wide range of topics, including sexual anatomy, reproductive health, psychological well-being, and the social dynamics of sexual relationships. Below, we delve into key theoretical frameworks, prevalent issues, and exemplary texts that contribute to a comprehensive understanding of sexual health and wellness.

Theoretical Frameworks

Understanding sexual health requires a multidisciplinary approach that incorporates psychology, sociology, medicine, and education. One prominent framework is the **Bio-Psycho-Social Model**, which posits that health is influenced by biological, psychological, and social factors. This model emphasizes that:

$$\text{Health} = f(\text{Biological Factors, Psychological Factors, Social Factors}) \quad (29)$$

This equation suggests that to achieve optimal sexual health, one must consider not only physical health (e.g., sexually transmitted infections, reproductive health) but also psychological well-being (e.g., anxiety, self-esteem) and social contexts (e.g., relationship dynamics, cultural norms).

Key Issues in Sexual Health

Several pressing issues emerge in the literature on sexual health and wellness, including:

- **Sexually Transmitted Infections (STIs):** The prevalence of STIs remains a significant concern. Education on prevention, testing, and treatment is crucial. Studies indicate that regular screening and open communication about sexual history can significantly reduce transmission rates.

- **Consent and Coercion:** Understanding the nuances of consent is vital. Research shows that many individuals struggle with asserting their boundaries, leading to potential coercion. Literature emphasizes the importance of clear communication and affirmative consent practices.

- **Body Image and Self-Esteem:** Body image issues can profoundly affect sexual health. The literature highlights that individuals with positive body image are more likely to engage in healthy sexual practices. Interventions aimed at improving self-esteem can enhance sexual experiences.

- **Access to Sexual Health Services:** Disparities in access to sexual health services can lead to negative health outcomes. Studies reveal that marginalized communities often face barriers to accessing comprehensive sexual health education and medical care.

Examples of Influential Texts

Numerous texts contribute to the discourse on sexual health and wellness. Here are a few notable examples:

- **"The Guide to Getting It On" by Paul Joannides:** This comprehensive guide covers a wide range of topics, from anatomy to techniques, emphasizing the importance of consent and communication in sexual encounters. It serves as an excellent resource for individuals seeking to enhance their sexual experiences while prioritizing health and wellness.

- **"Come as You Are" by Emily Nagoski:** This book delves into the science of sexual response and the impact of societal norms on sexual behavior. Nagoski's work encourages readers to embrace their sexuality and understand the factors that contribute to sexual well-being.

- **"Sexual Fluidity" by Lisa Diamond:** Diamond's research challenges traditional notions of sexual orientation, presenting a nuanced understanding of sexual desire and identity. Her work emphasizes the importance of recognizing the fluid nature of sexuality in fostering healthy relationships.

- **"The New Naked: The Ultimate Sex Education for Grown-Ups" by Harry Fisch:** This book offers a straightforward discussion on sexual health, addressing common myths and providing practical advice for maintaining sexual wellness throughout life.

Conclusion

Literature on sexual health and wellness provides invaluable insights into the complexities of human sexuality. By engaging with this body of work, individuals can better understand the interplay of biological, psychological, and social factors that influence their sexual experiences. As we explore breeding scenes and the erotic lifestyle, grounding our practices in a solid understanding of sexual health will enhance our experiences and foster deeper connections with partners.

Incorporating knowledge from this literature not only enriches our personal journeys but also empowers us to advocate for healthier sexual practices within our communities, ultimately leading to a more informed and fulfilling erotic lifestyle.

Erotic Fiction for Breeding Inspiration

Erotic fiction serves as a powerful medium for exploring desires, fantasies, and the intricate dynamics of breeding scenes. It allows readers to immerse themselves in narratives that evoke arousal and curiosity, providing a canvas for the imagination to run wild. In this section, we will delve into the significance of erotic fiction in the context of breeding, discuss various themes and tropes, and offer recommendations for literature that can ignite inspiration for your own breeding experiences.

The Role of Erotic Fiction in Sexual Exploration

Erotic fiction has long been a tool for sexual exploration, offering a safe space for individuals to confront their fantasies and desires. The narratives often encourage readers to reflect on their own experiences and preferences, fostering a deeper understanding of their sexuality. In the context of breeding scenes, erotic fiction can provide insights into the emotional and physical dynamics at play, helping readers navigate their own desires.

$$E = \frac{1}{2}mv^2 \tag{30}$$

In this equation, E represents the energy of sexual arousal, which can be influenced by various factors such as emotional connection (m) and the intensity of physical stimulation (v). Just as kinetic energy can be transformed and manipulated, so too can the energy of desire be cultivated through the narratives found in erotic fiction.

Common Themes in Breeding Erotica

Breeding erotica often incorporates several recurring themes that resonate with readers. Understanding these themes can enhance your appreciation of the genre and inspire your own creative endeavors. Here are some prevalent themes found in breeding fiction:

- **Desire for Fertility:** Many breeding stories explore the primal urge to procreate, tapping into deep-seated biological instincts. The characters may embody a longing for connection and the fulfillment that comes from creating life.

- **Power Dynamics:** The interplay of dominance and submission often features prominently in breeding scenes. Characters may navigate complex power structures, enhancing the tension and excitement of the narrative.

- **Forbidden Encounters:** Breeding erotica frequently delves into taboo relationships, such as those between family members, friends, or authority figures. These narratives evoke a thrill that stems from societal boundaries being crossed.

- **Community and Connection:** Many breeding stories emphasize the importance of community and shared experiences. Characters may engage in group breeding scenarios, highlighting the bonds formed through mutual desires.

- **Fantasy vs. Reality:** Breeding fiction often blurs the lines between fantasy and reality, inviting readers to explore scenarios that may not be feasible in their own lives. This exploration can lead to a greater understanding of personal desires and boundaries.

Recommended Reading for Breeding Inspiration

To assist you on your journey of exploration, here is a curated list of erotic fiction that focuses on breeding themes. These works not only entertain but also provide valuable insights into the dynamics of breeding scenes:

1. **"The Breeder's Club" by Amber Creame** - This novel offers a tantalizing glimpse into a secret society where breeding is celebrated. The characters navigate their desires in a world that embraces multiple partners and the joy of procreation.

2. **"Fertile Ground" by J. A. Black** - A story that explores the emotional complexities of a couple's journey to conceive. The narrative intertwines intimacy and the longing for family, creating a rich tapestry of desire.

3. **"The Alpha's Claim" by K. L. Hughes** - This paranormal romance delves into the world of werewolves, where breeding is tied to power and legacy. The

characters must navigate their instincts and emotions, leading to a gripping exploration of dominance and submission.

4. **"Breeding Season"** by L. D. Chase - Set in a dystopian future, this novel examines societal norms surrounding breeding. The characters' struggles against oppressive systems highlight the importance of choice and consent in breeding scenarios.

5. **"Taboo Desires"** by M. A. Sinclair - This collection of short stories features various taboo breeding scenarios, each exploring the thrill of forbidden encounters. The narratives challenge societal norms while celebrating the complexities of desire.

Writing Your Own Breeding Fiction

If you're inspired to create your own breeding narratives, consider the following tips to craft compelling and engaging stories:

- **Develop Rich Characters:** Create multidimensional characters with distinct motivations, desires, and backgrounds. This depth will enhance the emotional connection between the characters and the reader.

- **Explore Emotional Dynamics:** Focus on the emotional aspects of breeding scenes, such as vulnerability, trust, and intimacy. Highlighting these elements can elevate the tension and resonance of your narrative.

- **Incorporate Sensory Details:** Use vivid descriptions to engage the reader's senses. Paint a picture of the environment, the characters' physical sensations, and the emotional atmosphere to create a more immersive experience.

- **Challenge Stereotypes:** Push the boundaries of conventional breeding narratives by exploring diverse relationships and power dynamics. This can lead to innovative storytelling and a broader representation of desires.

- **Emphasize Consent and Communication:** Ensure that your characters engage in open communication and establish consent. This not only reflects healthy practices but also enhances the realism of your narrative.

In conclusion, erotic fiction serves as a vital resource for those seeking inspiration in breeding scenes. By exploring the themes and narratives within this genre, readers can gain a deeper understanding of their own desires and the dynamics of intimacy. Whether you choose to indulge in existing literature or create your own stories, the world of breeding erotica offers endless possibilities for exploration and connection.

Historical and Cultural References to Breeding

The concept of breeding, particularly in a sexual and erotic context, is steeped in historical and cultural significance. Throughout history, various societies have engaged in practices that reflect their views on sexuality, reproduction, and the roles of men and women in these processes. This section explores the multifaceted historical and cultural references to breeding, examining how these perspectives have evolved and influenced contemporary breeding scenes.

Ancient Civilizations and Fertility Cults

In ancient civilizations, breeding was often linked to fertility and the continuation of lineage. Cultures such as the Egyptians, Greeks, and Romans celebrated fertility through various rituals and deities. For instance, the Egyptian goddess Isis was revered as a protector of motherhood and fertility. Rituals often involved sexual rites aimed at ensuring bountiful harvests and healthy offspring, as fertility was crucial for agricultural societies.

$$F_{\text{fertility}} = C \cdot H \cdot R \tag{31}$$

Where:

- $F_{\text{fertility}}$ is the fertility rate.
- C is the cultural significance placed on fertility.
- H is the health of the community.
- R is the resources available for child-rearing.

This equation illustrates how various factors contribute to the perceived fertility of a society, emphasizing the connection between breeding and cultural values.

Medieval and Renaissance Perspectives

During the Medieval period in Europe, breeding was often viewed through the lens of marriage and property. The primary purpose of marriage was to produce heirs, and thus, breeding became a matter of social and economic importance. The concept of courtly love emerged, where romantic relationships were often idealized, yet the expectation remained that these unions would produce legitimate offspring.

In the Renaissance, a shift occurred as humanism began to influence thoughts on sexuality and reproduction. The focus on individual pleasure and the body led to a more open discussion about sexual desires. Artists and writers explored themes of breeding and sexuality, often blending eroticism with philosophical inquiries into human nature.

Colonial and Post-Colonial Perspectives

The colonial era introduced complex dynamics surrounding breeding, particularly in relation to power and control. Colonizers often imposed their own ideals of sexuality and reproduction on indigenous populations, resulting in a clash of cultural practices. The control over breeding rights became a method of exerting dominance, as seen in the forced breeding of enslaved individuals in the Americas.

Post-colonial discourse examines how these historical injustices continue to impact contemporary views on breeding and sexuality. The reclamation of cultural practices surrounding breeding has become a form of resistance against colonial narratives, allowing marginalized communities to redefine their identities and relationships with sexuality.

Modern Cultural References

In contemporary society, breeding has taken on new meanings, often influenced by media, literature, and sexual subcultures. The rise of erotic literature, particularly in the genre of BDSM and kink, has brought breeding scenes into the limelight. Authors like Anaïs Nin and contemporary writers have explored breeding as a means of expressing desire, power dynamics, and intimacy.

Cultural references in films, television, and online platforms have also contributed to the normalization of breeding scenes. The portrayal of breeding in popular culture often oscillates between romanticized ideals and raw, primal urges, reflecting society's complex relationship with sexuality.

Theoretical Perspectives on Breeding

Several theoretical frameworks can be applied to understand the cultural significance of breeding:

- **Feminist Theory:** Explores how breeding intersects with gender roles and power dynamics, emphasizing the need for consent and agency in reproductive choices.

- **Queer Theory:** Challenges traditional notions of breeding and sexuality, advocating for diverse expressions of desire that transcend heteronormative frameworks.

- **Psychoanalytic Theory:** Examines the unconscious motivations behind breeding desires, linking them to primal instincts and societal conditioning.

These perspectives highlight the complexity of breeding as a cultural phenomenon, revealing the interplay between individual desires and societal norms.

Conclusion

The historical and cultural references to breeding illustrate a rich tapestry of beliefs, practices, and theoretical frameworks that inform contemporary breeding scenes. By understanding these contexts, individuals can better appreciate the depth of their desires and the significance of breeding in their erotic lifestyles. As we continue to explore and experiment with breeding, it is essential to remain mindful of the historical narratives that shape our understanding of sexuality and reproduction.

Academic and Scientific Research on Various Aspects of Breeding

The exploration of breeding scenes, particularly within erotic contexts, has garnered increasing attention from both academic and scientific communities. This section aims to delve into the theoretical frameworks, empirical studies, and psychological implications surrounding breeding, emphasizing the multifaceted nature of this practice.

1. Theoretical Frameworks

Research on breeding can be understood through various theoretical lenses, including evolutionary psychology, sexual selection theory, and social constructivism.

1.1 Evolutionary Psychology From an evolutionary perspective, breeding behaviors can be linked to reproductive strategies aimed at maximizing genetic fitness. According to [?], individuals may engage in breeding scenes as a means of signaling fertility and desirability to potential mates. This is supported by the concept of *sexual selection*, which posits that traits enhancing mating success are favored over time.

The equation governing reproductive success can be expressed as:

$$R = \frac{(N_f \cdot S_f) + (N_m \cdot S_m)}{T} \tag{32}$$

where:

- R = reproductive success
- N_f = number of female partners
- S_f = success rate with female partners
- N_m = number of male partners
- S_m = success rate with male partners
- T = total time period of breeding activity

This equation highlights the balance between quantity and quality of mating opportunities, which can be particularly relevant in breeding scenes.

1.2 Sexual Selection Theory The sexual selection theory, as proposed by [?], posits that certain traits evolve not solely for survival but for attracting mates. This theory can be applied to breeding scenes, where the dynamics of power, attraction, and desirability play crucial roles. For instance, individuals may choose partners based on perceived genetic advantages, such as physical attributes or behavioral traits that signal health and vitality.

2. Empirical Studies

Several empirical studies have explored the psychological and sociological dimensions of breeding scenes.

2.1 Psychological Implications Research by [?] indicates that individuals who engage in breeding scenes often report heightened levels of intimacy and connection with their partners. This phenomenon can be attributed to the release of oxytocin, known as the "bonding hormone," which is associated with feelings of trust and emotional closeness.

2.2 Sociological Perspectives From a sociological standpoint, breeding scenes can be viewed through the lens of *social norms* and *cultural scripts*. A study by [?] found that societal attitudes towards breeding vary significantly across cultures, influencing how individuals express their desires and engage in breeding activities. For example, in cultures that emphasize family and reproduction, breeding scenes may be more openly accepted and celebrated.

3. Problems and Challenges

Despite the positive aspects associated with breeding scenes, several challenges and ethical considerations emerge in academic discussions.

3.1 Consent and Ethical Considerations The importance of consent is paramount in breeding scenes, as highlighted by [?]. The complexities of negotiating consent can lead to misunderstandings and potential harm if not navigated carefully. Researchers emphasize the need for clear communication and the establishment of boundaries to ensure all participants feel safe and respected.

3.2 Health Risks Health risks associated with breeding scenes, such as sexually transmitted infections (STIs) and unintended pregnancies, are critical areas of concern. A study by [?] underscores the necessity of safe practices, including the use of condoms and regular health check-ups, to mitigate these risks.

4. Examples of Research Applications

Practical applications of research findings can enhance the breeding experience for individuals. For instance, understanding the role of foreplay and its impact on sexual arousal can lead to more fulfilling breeding scenes. Research by [?] indicates that extended foreplay significantly enhances the likelihood of multiple orgasms, which is often a desired outcome in breeding scenarios.

5. Conclusion

In conclusion, the academic and scientific exploration of breeding scenes reveals a rich tapestry of psychological, sociological, and biological factors at play. As individuals navigate their desires within this erotic landscape, grounding their experiences in research can foster safer, more fulfilling encounters. Continued dialogue and inquiry into these aspects will not only enhance personal experiences but also contribute to a broader understanding of human sexuality.

Online Communities and Support Groups

Finding Like-Minded Individuals

In the pursuit of a breeding lifestyle, connecting with like-minded individuals can enhance your experiences, provide support, and foster a sense of community. This section explores various avenues for finding others who share your interests and desires, while also addressing potential challenges and solutions.

Understanding the Importance of Community

The need for connection is a fundamental aspect of human nature, often amplified within niche lifestyles such as breeding. Engaging with others who share similar interests can lead to:

- **Shared Knowledge:** Exchanging experiences and insights can enhance your understanding of breeding dynamics and techniques.

- **Emotional Support:** A community can offer encouragement and validation, particularly when navigating the complexities of alternative lifestyles.

- **Safety in Numbers:** Finding a group of like-minded individuals can create a safer environment for exploring your desires and fantasies.

Online Platforms and Communities

The internet provides a plethora of platforms where individuals can connect with others interested in breeding scenes. Here are some popular options:

- **Social Media Groups:** Platforms such as Facebook and Reddit host numerous groups dedicated to breeding and related lifestyles. Engaging in these communities can facilitate discussions, share experiences, and find partners.

- **Forums and Discussion Boards:** Websites like FetLife cater to various alternative lifestyles, including breeding. Users can post questions, share stories, and connect with others based on specific interests.

- **Dating Apps:** Specialized dating apps for kink and alternative lifestyles, such as KinkD and BDSM.com, allow users to filter potential partners based on their interests, including breeding.

Local Meetups and Events

In addition to online interactions, local meetups can provide opportunities to meet like-minded individuals in person. Consider the following:

- **Workshops and Classes:** Many cities host workshops focused on BDSM, sexuality, and alternative lifestyles. Participating in these events can help you meet individuals who share your interests while expanding your knowledge.

- **Social Events and Parties:** Attending local kink events, such as munches (casual meetups in public spaces) or private parties, can provide a relaxed environment to connect with others.

- **Community Centers:** Some cities have community centers dedicated to alternative lifestyles, offering regular events, discussions, and resources for individuals interested in breeding and related topics.

Navigating Challenges in Finding Community

While the search for like-minded individuals can be rewarding, it may also present challenges. Here are some common issues and strategies to overcome them:

- **Safety Concerns:** When meeting individuals online, prioritize your safety. Arrange initial meetings in public places, inform a friend of your whereabouts, and trust your instincts. Consider using a safe word or signal to communicate discomfort during interactions.

- **Misunderstandings:** Not everyone will share the same understanding of breeding scenes. Clear communication about your desires, boundaries, and expectations is essential. Utilize open-ended questions to foster dialogue and understanding.

- **Stigma and Judgment:** Engaging in alternative lifestyles can sometimes lead to stigma. Surrounding yourself with supportive individuals and communities can help mitigate feelings of isolation or judgment.

Examples of Successful Connections

To illustrate the potential benefits of finding like-minded individuals, consider the following examples:

- **Online Friendships:** A member of a breeding forum shared their experiences with multiple loads, leading to a friendship with another member. They began collaborating on educational content, helping others navigate their desires while deepening their own understanding.

- **Local Workshops:** A couple attended a local workshop on BDSM techniques, where they met others interested in breeding. They formed a small group that regularly meets to discuss experiences, share tips, and explore their interests together.

- **Public Events:** Attending a munch allowed an individual to connect with others who shared their passion for breeding. This connection led to a trusted partner with whom they could explore their fantasies safely and consensually.

Conclusion

Finding like-minded individuals is a crucial aspect of embracing the breeding lifestyle. By utilizing online platforms, attending local events, and navigating potential challenges, you can cultivate a supportive community that enhances your experiences. Remember, the journey is as important as the destination; fostering connections can lead to profound personal growth and shared exploration of desires.

Virtual Networking and Education

In the digital age, virtual networking and education have become essential tools for individuals exploring the breeding lifestyle. The internet offers a plethora of platforms where like-minded individuals can connect, share experiences, and learn from one another. This section delves into the various avenues available for virtual networking, the importance of education in fostering a healthy breeding lifestyle, and the potential challenges that may arise in online interactions.

Finding Like-Minded Individuals

One of the most significant advantages of virtual networking is the ability to connect with others who share similar interests and desires. Online communities can be found on various platforms, including:

- **Social Media Groups:** Platforms like Facebook and Reddit host numerous groups dedicated to breeding and alternative lifestyles. These groups provide a space for members to share stories, ask questions, and offer support.

- **Forums and Discussion Boards:** Websites such as FetLife and specialized forums allow users to engage in discussions, post articles, and share resources related to breeding. These platforms often have sections dedicated to specific interests, making it easier to find relevant conversations.

- **Virtual Meetups:** Many communities organize virtual meetups using platforms like Zoom or Discord. These meetings can include workshops, Q&A sessions, and casual chats, fostering a sense of community and connection among participants.

Connecting with others can help individuals feel less isolated in their interests and encourage them to explore their desires more openly.

Education and Resources

Education is a crucial component of navigating the breeding lifestyle safely and consensually. Several online resources provide valuable information on various aspects of breeding, including:

- **Webinars and Workshops:** Many educators and organizations offer virtual workshops on topics such as consent, communication, and safety in breeding scenes. These sessions often feature expert speakers and provide opportunities for participants to ask questions and engage in discussions.

- **Online Courses:** Websites like Skillshare and Udemy offer courses on sexual health, BDSM practices, and relationship dynamics. These courses can help individuals deepen their understanding of the breeding lifestyle and develop skills for enhancing their experiences.

- **Podcasts and YouTube Channels:** Numerous podcasts and YouTube channels focus on alternative lifestyles, including breeding. These platforms often feature interviews with experts, personal stories, and discussions on relevant topics, making them accessible and engaging resources for learning.

By utilizing these educational resources, individuals can gain insights into best practices, discover new techniques, and enhance their overall experiences within the breeding lifestyle.

Challenges of Virtual Networking

While virtual networking offers numerous benefits, it is not without its challenges. Some common issues that may arise include:

- **Miscommunication:** The absence of non-verbal cues in online interactions can lead to misunderstandings. It is essential to communicate clearly and confirm understanding, especially when discussing sensitive topics.

- **Privacy Concerns:** Sharing personal experiences and desires online can raise privacy issues. Individuals should be mindful of the information they disclose and consider using pseudonyms or private accounts to protect their identities.

- **Navigating Toxicity:** Not all online communities are positive or supportive. Individuals may encounter negativity, judgment, or harassment. It is crucial to recognize when a community is not a good fit and seek out safer spaces that align with one's values.

Addressing these challenges requires a proactive approach, including setting personal boundaries, practicing self-care, and seeking support from trusted individuals when needed.

Conclusion

Virtual networking and education play a vital role in the breeding lifestyle, offering opportunities for connection, learning, and growth. By engaging with online communities and utilizing educational resources, individuals can enhance their experiences, foster deeper connections, and navigate the complexities of breeding scenes with confidence and care. As the digital landscape continues to evolve, so too will the possibilities for exploration and connection within the breeding lifestyle.

Sharing Experiences and Seeking Advice

In the realm of breeding scenes and the broader erotic lifestyle, sharing experiences and seeking advice from others can be a transformative process. This section delves into the importance of community engagement, the benefits of sharing personal stories, and strategies for seeking advice effectively.

The Value of Community Engagement

Engaging with a community of like-minded individuals fosters a sense of belonging and validation. When individuals share their experiences, they contribute to a collective knowledge base that can help others navigate similar situations. This communal sharing can alleviate feelings of isolation and provide reassurance that one's desires and experiences are valid.

ONLINE COMMUNITIES AND SUPPORT GROUPS

Building Trust Through Shared Experiences

When participants openly share their stories, they cultivate trust within the community. This trust is essential for creating a safe space where individuals feel comfortable discussing their desires, boundaries, and experiences. The act of storytelling can also provide insights into diverse perspectives, enhancing empathy among community members.

Common Problems in Sharing Experiences

While sharing experiences can be beneficial, several challenges may arise:

- **Fear of Judgment:** Many individuals may hesitate to share their experiences due to concerns about being judged or misunderstood. This fear can prevent open dialogue and hinder personal growth.

- **Misinformation:** Not all advice shared within communities is accurate or beneficial. It is crucial to discern credible sources from anecdotal experiences that may not apply universally.

- **Emotional Vulnerability:** Sharing intimate experiences can expose individuals to emotional vulnerability. It is essential to approach these discussions with sensitivity and awareness of others' feelings.

Effective Strategies for Seeking Advice

To maximize the benefits of sharing experiences and seeking advice, consider the following strategies:

1. **Choose the Right Platform:** Identify forums, social media groups, or local meetups that cater specifically to breeding lifestyles. Look for spaces that prioritize consent, respect, and inclusivity.

2. **Be Specific in Your Queries:** When seeking advice, articulate your questions clearly. Providing context about your experiences and what you hope to achieve can lead to more tailored and relevant responses.

3. **Practice Active Listening:** When others share their experiences, practice active listening. This involves fully engaging with their stories, asking clarifying questions, and reflecting on their insights. Active listening fosters deeper connections and encourages reciprocal sharing.

4. **Respect Boundaries:** Not everyone may be comfortable sharing their experiences. Always approach conversations with respect for others' boundaries and privacy. Consent is paramount in all discussions, especially those involving sensitive topics.

5. **Follow Up:** If someone offers advice or shares a valuable experience, consider following up with them. This can deepen the relationship and provide opportunities for further discussion and learning.

Examples of Sharing Experiences

Consider the following hypothetical scenarios that illustrate the power of sharing experiences:

- **Scenario 1:** A participant shares their journey of exploring breeding scenes for the first time. They discuss their initial fears and how they navigated consent with their partner. This story resonates with others who may have similar apprehensions, encouraging them to engage in open dialogue about their feelings.

- **Scenario 2:** A seasoned participant offers advice on managing multiple loads effectively. They share techniques that worked for them and how they communicated with their partners to enhance mutual satisfaction. This practical advice can serve as a guide for newcomers seeking to enhance their experiences.

Conclusion

Sharing experiences and seeking advice is a vital aspect of engaging with the breeding lifestyle community. By fostering open dialogue, building trust, and practicing effective communication strategies, individuals can enhance their understanding of breeding scenes, navigate challenges, and cultivate deeper connections with others. This shared journey not only enriches personal experiences but also contributes to the collective wisdom of the community, creating a supportive environment for all who seek to explore their desires.

Building a Supportive Community for Your Breeding Lifestyle

Creating a supportive community around your breeding lifestyle is essential for fostering open communication, sharing experiences, and enhancing your overall enjoyment of breeding scenes. A well-connected community can provide a safe space to explore desires, seek advice, and develop meaningful relationships with like-minded individuals. In this section, we will explore the foundations of building such a community, the challenges you may face, and practical examples of how to cultivate these connections.

The Importance of Community

The need for community arises from our inherent social nature. Humans thrive on connection, and engaging with others who share similar interests can enhance our experiences. According to *Maslow's Hierarchy of Needs*, social belonging is a crucial aspect of human fulfillment. When it comes to breeding lifestyles, a supportive community can:

- Provide a safe environment for sharing fantasies and experiences.
- Offer emotional support and validation.
- Facilitate learning and personal growth through shared knowledge.
- Create opportunities for participation in group events and activities.

Challenges in Building Community

While the benefits of community are clear, there are challenges to consider. These may include:

- **Stigma and Misunderstanding:** Breeding lifestyles can be misunderstood or stigmatized by those outside the community. This can lead to fears of judgment or discrimination.
- **Diverse Perspectives:** Within the breeding community, individuals may have varying beliefs, practices, and desires, which can sometimes lead to conflict or discomfort.
- **Safety Concerns:** Ensuring a safe and consensual environment is paramount. The risk of encountering individuals who do not respect boundaries can create anxiety.

Strategies for Building Community

To overcome these challenges and foster a supportive breeding community, consider the following strategies:

1. **Establish Clear Communication Channels**   Creating dedicated platforms for discussion, such as online forums, social media groups, or chat applications, can facilitate open communication. Ensure these platforms are moderated to maintain a respectful and safe environment.

2. **Host Regular Meetups and Events**   Organizing events, whether in-person or virtual, allows community members to connect on a deeper level. These could include workshops, discussion groups, or social gatherings. For example, hosting a "Breeding 101" workshop can educate newcomers while reinforcing community bonds.

3. **Foster Inclusivity and Respect**   Encourage an inclusive atmosphere where all voices are heard and respected. This can involve setting ground rules for discussions, emphasizing the importance of consent, and being mindful of diverse perspectives within the community.

4. **Share Resources and Knowledge**   Create a repository of resources, including articles, books, and videos related to breeding lifestyles. Encourage members to contribute their favorite resources, fostering a culture of sharing and learning. This can be done via a community website or a shared document.

5. **Offer Support and Mentorship**   Establish mentorship programs where experienced community members can guide newcomers. This not only helps individuals navigate their desires but also strengthens the community as a whole. For instance, pairing a seasoned participant with someone new to the lifestyle can enhance their confidence and understanding.

6. **Utilize Online Platforms**   Leverage online platforms such as FetLife, Reddit, or specialized forums to connect with others interested in breeding. These platforms can help you find local groups, events, and discussions tailored to your interests.

Examples of Successful Communities

Several examples illustrate how supportive communities can thrive:

- **Local BDSM Clubs:** Many cities have BDSM clubs that host events focused on various kinks, including breeding. These clubs often prioritize education and consent, providing a safe space for exploration.

- **Online Forums:** Websites like FetLife allow users to create groups centered around specific interests, such as breeding. These groups can facilitate discussions, share experiences, and organize meetups.

- **Workshops and Retreats:** Organizations that focus on sexual wellness often offer workshops and retreats that delve into breeding dynamics, allowing participants to learn in a supportive environment.

Conclusion

Building a supportive community for your breeding lifestyle is a rewarding endeavor that can enrich your experiences and foster lasting connections. By prioritizing communication, inclusivity, and shared knowledge, you can create a vibrant community that celebrates and supports individual desires. Embrace the journey of connecting with others, and let the power of community enhance your breeding adventures.

Engaging with Online Workshops and Webinars

In the evolving landscape of the erotic lifestyle, online workshops and webinars have emerged as invaluable resources for individuals seeking to deepen their understanding and enhance their experiences, particularly within the realm of breeding scenes. These virtual platforms not only provide education but also foster a sense of community and connection among participants.

The Value of Online Learning

Participating in online workshops and webinars offers several key benefits:

- **Access to Expertise:** Many workshops are led by experienced educators, sexologists, and practitioners who specialize in various aspects of breeding and erotic lifestyles. This access to knowledgeable instructors can provide insights that may not be available through traditional reading materials.

- **Interactive Learning:** Unlike static resources, online workshops often include interactive components such as Q&A sessions, breakout discussions, and live demonstrations. This engagement allows participants to clarify doubts and explore topics in depth.

- **Anonymity and Comfort:** For those who may feel apprehensive about discussing intimate topics in person, online platforms provide a level of anonymity and comfort. Participants can engage from the safety of their homes, which can encourage more open dialogue.

- **Diverse Perspectives:** Online workshops attract participants from various backgrounds and experiences, creating a rich tapestry of perspectives. This diversity can lead to more comprehensive discussions and a broader understanding of breeding scenes.

Choosing the Right Workshop

When selecting an online workshop or webinar, consider the following factors:

- **Reputation of the Instructor:** Research the background and qualifications of the facilitator. Look for reviews or testimonials from previous participants to gauge the quality of the workshop.

- **Content Relevance:** Ensure that the topics covered align with your interests and goals. For example, if you are particularly interested in the dynamics of consent in breeding scenes, seek out workshops that emphasize this aspect.

- **Format and Duration:** Consider the format (live vs. recorded) and duration of the workshop. Some individuals may prefer shorter sessions, while others may benefit from extended workshops that allow for deeper exploration of topics.

- **Cost and Accessibility:** Evaluate the cost of the workshop and whether it fits within your budget. Some organizations offer sliding scale fees or scholarships to increase accessibility.

Popular Topics for Workshops

Online workshops can cover a wide range of topics relevant to breeding scenes. Some popular themes include:

- **Communication and Consent:** Workshops focusing on the nuances of consent, negotiation techniques, and establishing boundaries can empower participants to engage in breeding scenes safely and confidently.

- **Techniques for Maximizing Pleasure:** Sessions that delve into specific techniques for enhancing pleasure, such as the art of edging, prostate stimulation, and incorporating sensory experiences, can provide practical skills for participants.

- **Exploring Power Dynamics:** Workshops that examine the intersection of breeding scenes and power dynamics, including dominance and submission, can help participants navigate their roles and desires within these frameworks.

- **Safety and Health:** It is crucial to address health and safety concerns in breeding scenes. Workshops that cover sexual health, hygiene practices, and risk reduction strategies are essential for maintaining well-being.

- **Creative Roleplay and Fantasy:** Engaging in roleplay can enhance breeding experiences. Workshops that explore creative scenarios and character development can inspire participants to expand their imaginations.

Examples of Online Platforms

Several online platforms host workshops and webinars tailored to the erotic lifestyle community. Here are a few notable examples:

- **FetLife:** Known as a social networking site for the BDSM and kink community, FetLife often features announcements for workshops and educational events hosted by experienced practitioners.

- **Eventbrite:** This platform allows users to search for and register for various events, including workshops on erotic topics. Users can filter by location and interest to find relevant offerings.

- **Zoom:** Many independent educators and organizations utilize Zoom for hosting live workshops. Participants can join from anywhere in the world, making it a versatile option for learning.

- **YouTube:** While not a traditional workshop platform, many educators share valuable content through YouTube channels. These videos can serve as a supplement to formal workshops, providing additional insights and techniques.

Engaging with the Community

Beyond the educational aspects, online workshops and webinars offer an opportunity to connect with like-minded individuals. Engaging with fellow participants can lead to:

- **Networking Opportunities:** Building relationships with other attendees can enhance your support network and provide avenues for further exploration and collaboration in breeding scenes.

- **Shared Experiences:** Discussing personal experiences and insights with others can foster a sense of belonging and understanding within the community.

- **Collaborative Learning:** Participants can share resources, tips, and recommendations, enriching the learning experience for everyone involved.

Conclusion

Engaging with online workshops and webinars is an enriching way to enhance your understanding and experience of breeding scenes. By choosing the right workshops, actively participating, and connecting with others, you can deepen your knowledge and foster a sense of community within the erotic lifestyle. As you explore these educational opportunities, remember to approach each session with an open mind and a willingness to learn, allowing your breeding journey to flourish.

Professional Services

Therapists Specializing in Alternative Lifestyles

In the intricate world of breeding scenes and alternative lifestyles, the role of therapists who specialize in these areas cannot be overstated. These professionals provide a safe space for individuals to explore their desires, navigate complex emotions, and address any psychological barriers that may arise within their sexual experiences. This section will delve into the significance of seeking therapy, the common issues faced by individuals involved in alternative lifestyles, and the theoretical frameworks that underpin this therapeutic approach.

The Importance of Specialized Therapy

Therapists specializing in alternative lifestyles offer unique insights and support tailored to the specific needs of their clients. Unlike traditional therapists, who may lack an understanding of BDSM, kink, or breeding dynamics, these specialists are often well-versed in the psychological aspects of sexual expression. They provide guidance on how to navigate the emotional landscape of breeding scenes, including issues of consent, power dynamics, and the potential for emotional fallout.

PROFESSIONAL SERVICES

Common Issues Addressed in Therapy

Individuals engaging in breeding scenes may encounter several psychological challenges, including:

+ **Shame and Guilt:** Many individuals may struggle with feelings of shame or guilt regarding their desires, particularly if they come from backgrounds that stigmatize non-traditional sexual practices. Therapy can help in reframing these feelings and fostering self-acceptance.

+ **Communication Barriers:** Effective communication is crucial in any sexual relationship, especially in breeding scenes where consent and boundaries must be clearly established. Therapists can assist clients in developing better communication skills to express their desires and limits.

+ **Anxiety and Fear:** The intensity of breeding scenes can evoke anxiety or fear, particularly regarding the implications of such experiences (e.g., pregnancy, emotional attachment). Therapists can provide coping strategies and reassurance.

+ **Relationship Dynamics:** Breeding scenes often involve multiple partners, which can complicate relationship dynamics. Therapists can facilitate discussions around jealousy, trust, and emotional safety.

Theoretical Frameworks in Alternative Lifestyle Therapy

Therapists specializing in alternative lifestyles often draw from various theoretical frameworks to inform their practice. Some relevant theories include:

+ **Sexual Liberation Theory:** This framework emphasizes the importance of sexual expression as a fundamental human right. It advocates for the acceptance of diverse sexual practices and encourages individuals to embrace their desires without shame.

+ **Attachment Theory:** Understanding attachment styles can be crucial in breeding dynamics. Therapists may explore how clients' early relationships influence their current behaviors and emotional responses within breeding scenes.

+ **Cognitive Behavioral Therapy (CBT):** CBT can help clients identify and challenge negative thought patterns related to their sexual desires. By reframing these thoughts, individuals can cultivate a healthier relationship with their sexuality.

+ **Feminist Theory:** This perspective can be particularly relevant in discussions about power dynamics within breeding scenes. Therapists can help clients navigate issues of consent and autonomy, ensuring that all parties feel empowered in their choices.

Examples of Therapeutic Approaches

Therapists may employ various techniques to assist clients in exploring their breeding desires and addressing related issues:

+ **Role-Playing:** This technique allows clients to practice communication and boundary-setting in a safe environment. By simulating breeding scenarios, individuals can gain confidence in expressing their desires.

+ **Journaling:** Encouraging clients to maintain a journal can help them process their thoughts and feelings about their experiences. This practice can foster self-reflection and emotional awareness.

+ **Mindfulness and Grounding Techniques:** These strategies can help clients manage anxiety and stay present during intense experiences. Therapists may teach clients breathing exercises or visualization techniques to enhance their emotional regulation.

Finding the Right Therapist

When seeking a therapist specializing in alternative lifestyles, consider the following factors:

+ **Experience and Training:** Look for therapists who have specific training or certifications in sex therapy or alternative lifestyles. Their expertise will ensure they understand the nuances of breeding scenes.

+ **Comfort and Rapport:** A strong therapeutic alliance is essential for effective therapy. It's important to find a therapist with whom you feel comfortable discussing your desires and concerns.

+ **Approach and Philosophy:** Different therapists may employ various therapeutic approaches. Research potential therapists to find one whose philosophy aligns with your values and needs.

In conclusion, therapists specializing in alternative lifestyles play a vital role in supporting individuals exploring breeding scenes. By addressing common issues, employing relevant theoretical frameworks, and utilizing effective therapeutic techniques, these professionals can help clients navigate their desires and foster healthier relationships with their sexuality. Whether dealing with shame, communication barriers, or relationship dynamics, seeking specialized therapy can be a transformative step towards embracing one's breeding lifestyle.

Sex Educators and Coaches for Breeding Guidance

In the exploration of breeding scenes, the role of sex educators and coaches becomes paramount. These professionals provide invaluable insights, practical techniques, and emotional support tailored to individuals and couples interested in enhancing their breeding experiences. This section delves into the significance of seeking guidance from sex educators and coaches, the benefits they offer, and how to choose the right professional for your needs.

The Role of Sex Educators and Coaches

Sex educators and coaches specialize in various aspects of human sexuality, including but not limited to, communication techniques, sexual health, consent, and the intricacies of breeding dynamics. They can help individuals and couples navigate their desires and fantasies while ensuring that they do so in a safe, consensual, and informed manner.

Key Areas of Focus

- **Communication Skills:** Effective communication is the cornerstone of any successful breeding scene. Educators can teach techniques for expressing desires, setting boundaries, and negotiating consent. For instance, the use of "I" statements can help partners articulate their feelings and needs without placing blame or causing defensiveness.

- **Understanding Anatomy and Sexual Health:** Knowledge of anatomy is crucial for maximizing pleasure and ensuring safety during breeding scenes. Educators can provide information on male anatomy, the science of multiple orgasms, and safe practices to prevent sexually transmitted infections (STIs).

- **Emotional Intelligence:** The emotional aspects of breeding cannot be overlooked. Coaches can guide individuals in understanding their emotional responses to breeding scenes, including potential feelings of vulnerability or intimacy. This understanding is essential for fostering a safe and trusting environment.

+ **Techniques for Breeding Scenes:** From foreplay to aftercare, sex educators can offer a wealth of practical techniques to enhance the breeding experience. They may introduce various methods for maximizing pleasure, such as the art of edging, prostate stimulation, and the incorporation of roleplay.

+ **Safety and Consent:** Educators emphasize the importance of consent and safety in breeding scenes. They can help partners establish clear consent protocols, including the use of safewords and ongoing consent checks throughout the experience.

Common Problems Addressed by Educators

Individuals and couples may encounter several challenges when exploring breeding scenes. Sex educators and coaches can assist in addressing these issues:

+ **Communication Barriers:** Many couples struggle with openly discussing their desires and boundaries. Educators can facilitate conversations that break down these barriers and promote a healthier dialogue.

+ **Performance Anxiety:** Concerns about performance can detract from the enjoyment of breeding scenes. Coaches can provide strategies to alleviate anxiety, such as mindfulness techniques and focusing on the pleasure of the moment rather than outcomes.

+ **Navigating Emotional Triggers:** Breeding scenes can evoke strong emotional responses. Educators can help individuals identify their triggers and develop coping strategies to navigate these feelings effectively.

+ **Establishing Consent:** Misunderstandings about consent can lead to discomfort or harm. Educators can clarify what consent looks like in breeding scenarios and teach techniques for ensuring that all parties feel safe and respected.

Choosing the Right Educator or Coach

Selecting the right sex educator or coach is essential for a fulfilling learning experience. Consider the following factors:

- **Specialization:** Look for educators who specialize in breeding dynamics or related areas. Their expertise will ensure that the guidance you receive is relevant and applicable.

- **Approachability:** A good educator should create a safe and non-judgmental space for discussion. Feel free to ask about their teaching style and philosophy before committing.

- **Credentials and Experience:** Verify the educator's qualifications and experience. Professional certifications from recognized organizations can indicate a level of expertise and commitment to ethical practices.

- **Client Testimonials:** Seek feedback from previous clients to gauge the effectiveness of the educator's methods and the overall experience.

- **Compatibility:** Personal compatibility is crucial. A strong rapport with your educator will enhance your learning experience and foster trust.

Conclusion

Engaging with sex educators and coaches can significantly enrich your breeding journey. Their expertise can illuminate the complexities of breeding scenes, empower you with knowledge, and help you navigate challenges with confidence. By investing in your education, you not only enhance your own experiences but also contribute to a culture of informed and consensual exploration within the breeding lifestyle.

Medical Experts for Sexual Health and Wellness

In the realm of erotic lifestyles, particularly those involving breeding scenes, the importance of consulting with medical experts cannot be overstated. These professionals provide crucial insights into sexual health, wellness, and safety, ensuring that individuals can explore their desires without compromising their physical or emotional well-being.

Understanding Sexual Health

Sexual health is a multifaceted aspect of overall health that encompasses physical, emotional, mental, and social well-being in relation to sexuality. The World Health Organization (WHO) defines sexual health as:

"...a state of physical, emotional, mental, and social well-being in relation to sexuality; it is not merely the absence of disease, dysfunction, or infirmity."

This definition highlights the need for a holistic approach to sexual health, especially in contexts that involve intimate and often vulnerable experiences, such as breeding scenes.

The Role of Medical Experts

Medical experts, including sex therapists, gynecologists, urologists, and sexual health educators, play a pivotal role in providing guidance and support in the following areas:

- **Sexual Health Assessments:** Regular check-ups can help identify any potential health issues that may affect sexual performance or pleasure. This includes screenings for sexually transmitted infections (STIs), hormonal assessments, and evaluations of reproductive health.

- **Safe Practices:** Medical professionals can educate individuals about safe sexual practices, including the use of condoms and dental dams, which are essential for preventing STIs and ensuring a healthy breeding experience.

- **Fertility Awareness:** For those interested in breeding, understanding fertility cycles is vital. Medical experts can provide information on ovulation tracking and the optimal times for conception, enhancing the breeding experience.

- **Addressing Concerns:** Individuals may experience anxiety or concerns regarding their sexual health. Medical experts can offer counseling and support, addressing issues such as performance anxiety, sexual dysfunction, and emotional well-being.

Common Health Issues in Breeding Scenes

When engaging in breeding scenes, individuals may encounter several health-related issues, including but not limited to:

- **Sexually Transmitted Infections (STIs):** The risk of STIs increases with multiple partners. Regular testing and open communication about sexual history are essential.

PROFESSIONAL SERVICES 203

- **Hormonal Imbalances:** Hormonal fluctuations can impact libido and sexual function. Consulting with an endocrinologist can help address these issues.

- **Reproductive Health Issues:** Conditions such as polycystic ovary syndrome (PCOS) or endometriosis can affect fertility and overall sexual health. Gynecologists can provide treatment options and management strategies.

Consultation Examples

To illustrate the importance of medical experts in sexual health, consider the following examples:

1. **Case Study: Fertility Counseling**
   A couple interested in breeding seeks the help of a fertility specialist. After a thorough assessment, the specialist recommends lifestyle changes, such as diet and exercise, and provides information on ovulation tracking. This guidance increases the couple's chances of conception and enhances their breeding experience.

2. **Case Study: STI Awareness**
   An individual engaging in group breeding scenes consults with a sexual health educator about STI risks. The educator provides information on safe sex practices and emphasizes the importance of regular testing. This knowledge empowers the individual to make informed decisions and protect their health.

Finding the Right Medical Expert

When seeking medical experts for sexual health and wellness, consider the following steps:

- **Research:** Look for professionals with experience in sexual health, reproductive health, and alternative lifestyles. Online reviews and professional associations can provide valuable information.

- **Consultation:** Schedule an initial consultation to discuss your specific needs and concerns. This meeting can help determine if the expert is a good fit for your situation.

- **Ongoing Communication:** Maintain open lines of communication with your medical expert. Regular check-ins can help address any emerging concerns and ensure that you are on the right track.

Conclusion

Incorporating the insights of medical experts into your erotic lifestyle can significantly enhance your experiences, particularly in breeding scenes. By prioritizing sexual health and wellness, individuals can explore their desires with confidence, ensuring that their journeys are both pleasurable and safe. Remember, your health is paramount—never hesitate to seek professional guidance when navigating the complexities of your erotic lifestyle.

Adult Toy and Accessories Suppliers

In the realm of breeding scenes, the right tools and accessories can significantly enhance the experience, creating an environment ripe for exploration and pleasure. This section delves into the various types of adult toys and accessories that can complement breeding activities, as well as reputable suppliers that cater to these specific needs.

Types of Adult Toys for Breeding Scenes

1. **Vibrators and Dildos**: These are staples in any erotic lifestyle. Vibrators can be used for clitoral stimulation, while dildos can simulate penetration. For breeding scenes, consider toys that are designed to mimic the sensations of fullness and stimulation that accompany breeding. Some dildos come with realistic textures and shapes that enhance the experience.

2. **Cock Rings**: These accessories can help prolong erections and enhance pleasure for the wearer. By constricting blood flow, cock rings can lead to increased stamina and intensity during breeding scenes. Look for adjustable options to ensure comfort and safety.

3. **Prostate Massagers**: For those interested in exploring prostate stimulation, specialized massagers can provide intense pleasure. These toys can help in achieving multiple orgasms, which is a key aspect of breeding dynamics.

4. **Paddles and Whips**: Incorporating elements of BDSM can heighten the intensity of breeding scenes. Paddles and whips can be used to establish power dynamics, adding an exciting layer of anticipation and submission to the experience.

5. **Restraints and Bondage Gear**: For couples looking to explore power dynamics, restraints can be a thrilling addition. Whether it's handcuffs, ropes, or harnesses, these tools can enhance the feeling of surrender that many find exhilarating during breeding scenes.

6. **Breeding Kits**: Some suppliers offer specialized breeding kits that include a combination of toys designed to enhance breeding experiences. These kits may include items like vaginal balls, fertility-focused lubricants, and instructional guides.

Choosing the Right Suppliers

When selecting adult toys and accessories, it's vital to choose reputable suppliers who prioritize quality, safety, and customer service. Here are some considerations:

1. **Material Safety**: Ensure that the toys are made from body-safe materials such as silicone, glass, or stainless steel. Avoid products containing phthalates or other harmful chemicals.

2. **Reviews and Reputation**: Research suppliers by reading customer reviews and checking their reputation within the community. Websites that specialize in sexual wellness often provide detailed reviews and ratings.

3. **Return Policies and Customer Support**: A good supplier should offer a reasonable return policy and responsive customer support. This is crucial for ensuring satisfaction with your purchases.

4. **Discretion and Privacy**: Choose suppliers that respect your privacy and provide discreet shipping options. This is particularly important for those who may be exploring breeding scenes for the first time.

5. **Educational Resources**: Some suppliers go beyond selling products by offering educational resources, including guides on how to use specific toys, safety tips, and advice on enhancing your sexual experiences.

Recommended Suppliers

Here are a few reputable adult toy suppliers known for their quality products and excellent customer service:

1. **Lovehoney**: This supplier offers a wide range of adult toys, including those specifically designed for breeding scenes. They provide extensive product descriptions, customer reviews, and educational articles.

2. **Adam & Eve**: Known for their extensive selection and commitment to customer satisfaction, Adam & Eve offers a variety of toys suitable for breeding dynamics, including high-quality dildos and vibrators.

3. **SheVibe**: This supplier is known for its focus on body-safe materials and a diverse range of products. Their website features a user-friendly design and detailed product information.

4. **Babeland**: With a commitment to sexual health and wellness, Babeland offers a curated selection of toys and accessories, including educational resources that can enhance your breeding experience.

5. **EdenFantasys**: This supplier offers a wide variety of adult toys, including many that cater to breeding fantasies. They also provide a community forum where customers can share experiences and advice.

Conclusion

Incorporating adult toys and accessories into breeding scenes can elevate the experience, making it more enjoyable and fulfilling. By selecting the right tools and sourcing them from reputable suppliers, individuals can enhance their breeding adventures while ensuring safety and pleasure. Always prioritize communication with partners about preferences and boundaries when introducing new toys into your intimate encounters. As you explore the world of adult toys, remember that the journey of discovery is just as important as the destination, allowing for deeper connections and shared experiences.

Event Organizers and Party Planners for Breeding Gatherings

When it comes to hosting breeding gatherings, the role of event organizers and party planners is crucial in creating a safe, enjoyable, and fulfilling experience for all participants. This section delves into the various aspects of organizing such events, addressing potential challenges, and providing practical examples to ensure success.

Understanding the Role of Event Organizers

Event organizers are responsible for the logistics and overall atmosphere of breeding gatherings. Their tasks include:

- **Venue Selection:** Choosing a location that is both private and conducive to the activities planned. This could range from private homes to rented spaces that offer a sense of intimacy and security.

- **Theme Development:** Crafting a theme that resonates with the participants and enhances the experience. Themes can vary from sensual and romantic to more adventurous and playful.

- **Safety Protocols:** Establishing guidelines to ensure the safety and comfort of all attendees. This includes setting up safe words, consent protocols, and emergency contact systems.

PROFESSIONAL SERVICES   207

- **Resource Provision:** Providing necessary resources such as educational materials on safe practices, health information, and access to sexual wellness products.

Challenges in Organizing Breeding Gatherings

While organizing breeding gatherings can be rewarding, it also comes with its challenges. Some common issues include:

- **Consent Management:** Ensuring that all participants understand and respect consent is paramount. Organizers must implement clear communication strategies to facilitate this.

- **Diverse Participant Needs:** Attendees may have varying levels of experience and comfort with breeding scenes. Organizers should create an inclusive environment that caters to all.

- **Legal Considerations:** Depending on the location, there may be legal implications surrounding public displays of affection and sexual activities. It is essential to be aware of and adhere to local laws.

Strategies for Successful Event Planning

To navigate these challenges effectively, event organizers can employ several strategies:

1. **Pre-Event Surveys:** Distributing surveys to gauge participants' interests, comfort levels, and expectations can help tailor the event to meet their needs. This information can inform decisions regarding activities, themes, and safety measures.

2. **Workshops and Educational Sessions:** Incorporating workshops on topics such as consent, communication, and safe practices can enhance the experience and empower participants. These sessions can foster a sense of community and shared learning.

3. **Designated Safe Spaces:** Creating areas within the venue where attendees can retreat for a moment of privacy or to discuss boundaries can enhance comfort levels. These spaces should be clearly marked and accessible.

4. Experienced Staff: Hiring or recruiting knowledgeable staff who understand the dynamics of breeding gatherings can provide additional support and ensure that the event runs smoothly. This may include facilitators, security personnel, or health professionals.

Examples of Successful Breeding Gatherings

To illustrate effective event planning, here are a few examples of successful breeding gatherings:

Example 1: Themed Private Party A private gathering themed around "Sensual Harvest" brought together individuals interested in exploring breeding scenes. The organizers created an intimate atmosphere with dim lighting, soft music, and seasonal decor. Pre-event surveys helped tailor activities, which included guided discussions on desires and boundaries, followed by sensual activities that encouraged connection.

Example 2: Educational Retreat An educational retreat focused on breeding dynamics included workshops led by sex educators and experienced practitioners. Participants engaged in discussions about emotional well-being, consent, and techniques for enhancing pleasure. The event fostered a sense of community and provided a safe space for exploration.

Example 3: Public Play Party A well-organized public play party ensured safety and consent through the implementation of wristbands indicating consent levels. Attendees participated in various activities, including demonstrations and roleplay, while designated areas for discussion and aftercare were established.

Conclusion

Event organizers and party planners play a pivotal role in the success of breeding gatherings. By understanding the unique needs of participants, addressing potential challenges, and employing effective strategies, they can create memorable and fulfilling experiences. As the breeding lifestyle continues to evolve, the importance of skilled organizers in fostering safe and enjoyable environments cannot be overstated. Embracing these principles will not only enhance individual experiences but also contribute to the broader community's growth and acceptance of diverse sexual expressions.

Index

a, 1–6, 8–13, 15–25, 27–32, 34,
    37–45, 47–51, 53, 54,
    56–60, 62–67, 69–71,
    73–75, 77–83, 85, 87–89,
    92, 94–107, 109, 110, 112,
    113, 115, 117–120, 123,
    125–129, 131, 133–139,
    141–143, 145–159,
    161–167, 171, 173–181,
    183, 184, 186–196,
    198–203, 205, 206, 208
ability, 6, 43, 60, 69, 70, 74, 77, 79, 186
acceptance, 24, 150, 166, 208
accomplishment, 5
account, 23
act, 3–5, 15, 16, 18, 24, 47, 80, 95, 131, 153, 189
action, 155
activity, 23, 28, 40, 72, 73, 100
adaptability, 37, 162
addition, 81, 87, 184
adherence, 23
adult, 151, 204–206
adventure, 37, 95, 133, 157, 158, 163
advice, 1, 3, 89, 188–191
affirmation, 5
aftercare, 4, 9, 10, 12, 98, 115, 150, 160
afterthought, 150
age, 70, 186
agreement, 20, 21, 101, 119
aid, 77, 79
air, 42
alignment, 31
allure, 3, 5, 114, 129
ambiance, 11, 41, 42, 44, 48, 51, 52
Americas, 180
amount, 56
anatomy, 12, 58, 60, 69, 71, 74, 77, 174
Anaïs Nin, 180
anticipation, 63, 65, 80, 82
anxiety, 73, 79, 109, 146, 148, 150, 155
application, 57, 108
appreciation, 176
approach, 3, 4, 28, 30, 76, 95, 103, 118, 156, 160, 161, 188, 196, 202
archaeologist, 94
archive, 158
area, 42, 56
aromatherapy, 49
arousal, 6, 7, 11, 19, 37, 41–43, 46, 48–51, 54–56, 58–60, 64,

    65, 70, 73, 78, 80, 85, 87,
        88, 96, 129, 132, 133, 156,
        163, 176
array, 1
arrest, 130
art, 48, 51, 58, 65, 82
aspect, 5, 19, 20, 22, 25, 30, 37, 39,
        41, 62, 83, 101, 112, 118,
        129, 149, 156, 162, 184,
        186, 190
assessment, 118, 120, 126, 203
assistance, 147
association, 18
atmosphere, 24, 42, 43, 46, 48–52,
        54, 96, 113, 129, 137, 192,
        206
attachment, 18, 20, 22, 150, 151
attention, 4, 43, 51, 56, 134, 135,
        181
attentiveness, 104
attire, 94
attitude, 162
attraction, 42
attribute, 71
audience, 166
authority, 118
autonomy, 23, 99, 112, 127
avenue, 137
aversion, 23
awareness, 37, 79, 131, 132, 153

back, 31, 156
backdrop, 42, 50
background, 42
balance, 80, 136, 157, 158, 182
base, 59, 78, 188
basic, 19
bath, 149

BDSM, 19, 113, 115–117, 163, 171,
        173, 180, 196
beauty, 8
bedrock, 34
bedroom, 48
behavior, 18, 129, 134, 136
being, 4, 12, 13, 17, 32, 34, 97, 99,
        101, 132, 136, 142, 145,
        146, 148, 156–158, 161,
        174, 192, 201
belief, 24
belonging, 5, 8, 18, 188
benefit, 146
bladder, 70
blend, 116, 117, 132, 134
blindfold, 47, 94
bodily, 24, 79
body, 5, 6, 21, 56, 69–72, 77, 83,
        103, 149, 175, 179
bond, 9, 10, 12, 20, 24, 152
bonding, 9, 18, 47, 69, 150–152
boundary, 134, 135
breach, 30
breath, 57, 70
breathing, 70, 73, 85
breeder, 19
breeding, 3–5, 7–13, 15–25, 27,
        29–35, 37–46, 48–58,
        60–63, 65–67, 69, 71, 73,
        74, 77, 80–83, 86–101,
        103–113, 115–120,
        123–132, 134–139,
        141–143, 145, 146,
        148–164, 174–184,
        186–188, 190–194,
        196–204, 206–208
bridge, 141
brink, 80

Index 211

building, 63, 72, 82, 131, 137, 138, 164, 190, 191

calming, 42
candlelight, 42
canvas, 67, 176
capacity, 6, 72
care, 76, 92, 148, 150, 188
case, 74
catalyst, 8
celebration, 82
challenge, 3, 23, 25
change, 37, 102, 103, 162, 164
character, 48, 60, 92, 94
charge, 19
chat, 192
check, 101, 103, 119, 152
checkbox, 109
checklist, 157
choice, 42
clarity, 28, 31, 109, 148, 156, 162
clash, 180
climax, 64, 65
closeness, 150
coach, 200
coercion, 23
collar, 157
combination, 59, 71
comfort, 20, 38, 42–44, 46, 47, 50, 101, 110, 112, 129, 134, 136, 151
commitment, 10, 23–25, 34, 106, 109, 117, 120, 127, 158
communication, 4, 10, 11, 13, 18, 19, 21, 22, 24, 25, 28–30, 32–38, 40, 48, 57, 60, 62, 65, 82, 99, 101, 103, 104, 106, 109, 110, 112, 115, 117, 118, 120, 125, 126, 129, 131, 132, 135, 136, 139, 143, 152, 155–159, 161, 173, 190, 192, 193, 199, 206
community, 5, 16, 19, 24, 129, 131, 137–139, 150, 158, 163, 164, 183, 186, 188–193, 195, 196, 208
companion, 3
complexity, 22, 109, 111, 115, 181
component, 9, 12, 21, 28, 34, 40, 49, 60, 63, 71, 101, 141, 150, 153, 160, 174, 187
concept, 17, 18, 95, 113, 115, 179
conception, 15, 16, 203
concern, 59
conclusion, 5, 7, 18, 29, 46, 51, 77, 92, 98, 101, 106, 112, 120, 143, 155, 158, 161, 164, 178, 183, 199
conditioning, 71
conduct, 56, 127, 130, 136
confidence, 4, 94, 148, 156, 188, 192, 201
confidentiality, 30
confusion, 142
connection, 3–5, 8–10, 12, 15, 18, 20, 23, 24, 29, 32, 42, 47, 48, 50–52, 54, 62, 67, 69, 71, 74, 77, 79, 80, 83, 95–98, 104, 106, 117, 120, 123, 131, 137, 139, 145, 148, 150, 152, 156, 158, 164, 178, 179, 184, 188, 193
consent, 4, 9, 12, 13, 18–25, 32, 34, 48, 57, 62, 82, 101–104, 106–112, 116–120, 126, 129, 131, 132, 135, 136,

139, 143, 158, 173, 192, 196, 199
consideration, 51, 114, 129, 132, 139
contact, 56, 152
content, 2
context, 20, 27, 37, 46, 48, 69, 83, 104, 123, 126, 134, 176, 179
continuation, 3, 179
continuity, 152
contraception, 24
contrast, 57
control, 4, 19, 70, 73, 77–80, 113, 118, 123, 180
conversation, 31, 37, 100, 103, 118
core, 1, 3, 18, 69, 73, 80
cornerstone, 11, 28, 118, 135, 159
counter, 4
couple, 9, 23, 74, 103, 129, 157, 203
creation, 18
creativity, 48, 58, 60, 156
cuddling, 145, 149
culture, 109, 166, 180, 192, 201
curiosity, 176
customer, 205
cycle, 64, 65, 73, 77, 153, 154
cycling, 72

dance, 109
dancing, 72
debrief, 103
debriefing, 12, 39, 66, 141–143, 145
decency, 130
definition, 95, 202
degree, 136
denial, 80
depth, 65, 156, 181
desirability, 5

desire, 3, 11, 18–21, 23, 39, 42, 60, 63, 71, 164, 165, 180
destination, 32, 60, 67, 164, 186, 206
detail, 51
development, 92, 125
device, 87
dialogue, 4, 11, 28, 30–35, 37, 100, 101, 105, 143, 145, 147, 149, 151, 183, 190
diet, 203
difficulty, 85, 101
discomfort, 31, 34, 42, 110, 129, 135, 149, 155, 157, 159
discontent, 129
discourse, 4, 175, 180
discovery, 60, 67, 86, 126, 131, 150, 153, 156, 206
discretion, 136
discussing, 4, 28, 30, 40, 145, 149, 151, 189
discussion, 31, 38, 101, 135, 180, 192
distraction, 97
distress, 101, 160
diversity, 25, 165
document, 158, 192
dominance, 3, 19, 47, 115, 180
dominant, 4, 19, 23, 94, 103, 118, 123, 157
down, 24
drawing, 135, 150
drink, 149
drive, 3, 94
dynamic, 4, 22, 23, 37, 39, 47, 65, 94, 102, 104, 112, 113, 118, 123–126

ease, 28

ecstasy, 5
edge, 80
edging, 64, 65, 80–82
education, 158, 186, 188, 193, 201
educator, 200, 203
effect, 42
effectiveness, 28, 76
effort, 120
ejaculation, 70, 77–80
element, 18, 20, 56, 57, 106
emotion, 53
empathy, 10, 104, 106, 189
empowerment, 4, 5, 156
encounter, 2, 10, 11, 20–22, 24, 27, 37, 42, 63, 73, 85, 109, 141, 157, 158, 162, 197, 200, 202
encouragement, 163
end, 143, 161
endeavor, 51, 71, 136, 139, 193
endurance, 71, 73
engagement, 42, 46, 123, 188
enjoyment, 132, 190
enthusiasm, 9, 21
environment, 10–13, 19, 22, 24, 29, 31, 32, 34, 37, 40, 42, 43, 46, 48, 49, 51, 54, 60, 71, 92, 101, 104, 109, 112, 120, 128, 129, 132, 137, 138, 148, 151, 152, 155, 158, 160, 165, 166, 190, 192, 204
equation, 21, 80, 119, 130, 165, 179, 181, 182
era, 180
erotica, 176, 178
eroticism, 16, 60, 112, 180
essence, 3

establishing, 11, 19, 27–29, 41, 99, 101, 129, 136, 139, 150, 152, 157
establishment, 158
esteem, 5
euphoria, 148
Europe, 179
evening, 31
event, 129, 136, 206–208
example, 4, 9, 11, 24, 29, 31, 42, 54, 59, 70, 73, 84, 88, 129, 135, 149, 156, 157, 166
exchange, 23, 24, 113–116, 118, 120
excitement, 16, 65, 94, 109, 115, 134, 137, 146, 156, 163
exercise, 72, 153, 203
exhibitionism, 17
expectation, 179
experience, 1, 4, 5, 9–13, 17–20, 23, 24, 27, 29, 30, 32–34, 40, 42–44, 46–48, 55–57, 59, 60, 62, 63, 65, 69–71, 77, 79, 80, 83–89, 92, 94, 95, 97–99, 101, 102, 104, 106, 109, 112, 115–119, 123, 126–129, 133, 136, 137, 141–143, 145, 148–150, 152, 153, 155–158, 160, 164, 196, 200, 203, 204, 206
experiment, 62, 157, 158, 181
experimentation, 126, 156–158
expertise, 201
exploration, 1, 3–5, 8–10, 12, 13, 16, 20, 24, 27, 29, 32, 37, 48, 54, 60, 67, 77, 80, 83, 86, 92, 95, 109, 112, 117, 120, 123, 126, 131, 139, 152, 156, 158, 161, 163,

164, 166, 171, 174,
176–178, 181, 183, 186,
188, 199, 201, 204
exposure, 111
expression, 23, 24, 60, 62, 145, 150, 196
extent, 99
eye, 152

facet, 129
fallout, 196
fantasy, 3, 17, 18, 48, 60, 65, 67, 85, 96, 98, 163
fatigue, 59
fear, 19, 23, 24, 27, 30, 43, 100, 157
feedback, 4
feel, 4, 5, 10, 19–21, 24, 28, 30, 31, 37, 38, 42, 47, 48, 58, 62, 100, 101, 104, 105, 111, 118, 128, 141, 149, 151, 165, 166, 187, 189
feeling, 47, 103, 137, 155
fertility, 3, 18, 179, 203
FetLife, 192
fiction, 150, 176–178
figure, 94, 157
finding, 184, 185
flexibility, 37
floor, 31, 73, 78
fluid, 23, 75
fluidity, 126, 162
focus, 10, 40, 58, 70, 73, 79, 179
force, 18, 56
forefront, 161
foreplay, 63–65
form, 18, 24, 58, 180
foundation, 1, 10, 34, 107, 124, 158, 171

framework, 4, 23, 27, 30, 37, 107, 109, 127, 134
Freud, 18
friction, 56, 87
fulfillment, 3, 4, 8, 19, 164
function, 70
fusion, 115
future, 39, 40, 105, 154–156, 161, 163, 164

gathering, 24
gender, 23
genre, 176, 178, 180
gesture, 135
Gibbs, 154
gland, 70, 75
glass, 31
go, 99
goal, 79, 126
goddess, 179
grip, 84
ground, 192
group, 18, 23, 106–109, 111, 127–129, 155, 203
growth, 5, 24, 139, 153, 154, 158, 162, 163, 171, 186, 188, 208
guidance, 145, 148, 150, 196, 199, 202, 203
guide, 3, 10–13, 30, 48, 67, 106, 112, 129, 153, 156, 192
guilt, 85, 86, 142

hand, 16, 99, 135
harness, 96
haven, 48, 157
head, 78
healing, 145

Index 215

health, 24, 32–34, 38, 70, 72, 145, 148, 157, 158, 161, 166, 174–176, 199, 201–203
heart, 69, 72, 80
help, 19, 42, 70, 71, 73, 84, 85, 88, 101, 104, 124, 125, 145, 149–151, 154, 163, 187, 188, 192, 199, 201, 203
hesitation, 21
highlight, 181
history, 179
home, 31, 42
hormone, 18, 69
host, 195
hosting, 206
human, 1, 3, 18, 19, 42, 69, 71, 162, 175, 180, 183, 184, 199
humanism, 179
hydration, 59
hygiene, 88–92

ice, 57, 59
idea, 18, 31
ideal, 13, 45
identity, 5, 23
imagination, 48, 67, 176
impact, 5, 48, 60, 62, 79, 106, 180
importance, 5, 7, 11, 12, 20, 29, 30, 32, 34, 35, 37, 42, 43, 101, 103, 106, 118, 128, 129, 141, 148, 153, 155, 156, 160, 162, 165, 179, 186, 188, 192, 201, 203, 208
in, 1, 3–5, 7–13, 15, 18–24, 28–35, 37–44, 46, 48, 49, 51–53, 57, 59, 60, 63–67, 69–77, 79, 82, 83, 85, 87–90, 92, 94–104, 106–113, 115, 117–120, 123–137, 141, 143, 145, 146, 148–165, 173, 174, 176, 178–184, 186–188, 192, 193, 196–203, 206, 208
incense, 42
include, 1, 7, 9, 12, 16, 17, 29, 31, 38, 44, 46, 56, 58, 61, 70, 76, 97, 98, 100–102, 136, 137, 142, 145, 146, 149, 151, 152, 154, 159, 160, 165, 187, 191, 194, 197, 206, 207
inclusivity, 193
incorporating, 11, 12, 49, 57, 61, 80, 94, 95, 98, 133, 150–152, 155, 162, 163
incorporation, 46, 115, 116, 163
increase, 59, 70, 72, 73
indecency, 128, 136
individual, 78, 88, 99, 101, 109, 129, 139, 150, 179, 181, 193, 203, 208
individuality, 23
influence, 28, 42, 43, 48, 50, 52, 118, 151, 160, 175, 179
information, 30, 135, 187, 203
initiator, 4
inquiry, 183
insecurity, 19, 150, 152
insight, 18
inspiration, 163, 166, 176, 178
instance, 23, 24, 31, 42, 47, 60, 88, 100, 136, 150, 151, 156, 163, 179, 192
instinct, 3
integration, 51, 88
intensity, 40, 51, 59, 72, 73, 80, 82, 88, 116
intent, 15–17

intention, 58
interaction, 106, 134
intercourse, 15, 24
internet, 184, 186
interplay, 7, 19–21, 60, 71, 123, 175, 181
interruption, 43
intersection, 3
intertwine, 101, 148
interval, 73
intimacy, 3–5, 8–11, 15, 18, 20, 22–24, 27, 29, 30, 33, 34, 37, 39, 41–43, 47, 48, 50, 52, 54, 58, 77, 80, 95, 97–99, 101, 106, 113, 117, 126, 132, 133, 143, 145, 148, 150–152, 155, 158, 160, 164, 178, 180
intrigue, 3, 23
investment, 106
invitation, 1, 71
isolation, 188
issue, 66

jaw, 59
jazz, 42
jealousy, 19, 152
John Bowlby, 18
journal, 145, 158
journaling, 154
journey, 3, 7, 10, 13, 30, 32, 34, 37, 60, 67, 71, 77, 80, 82, 98, 104, 126, 131, 139, 143, 146, 153, 154, 156, 158, 161, 164, 177, 186, 190, 193, 196, 201, 206
joy, 163
judgment, 19, 23, 25, 30, 97, 100, 157

jurisdiction, 127

Kegel, 78, 80
key, 1, 18, 34, 48, 58, 64, 82, 87, 92, 110, 114, 116, 118, 120, 124, 129, 136, 141, 154, 171, 174, 193
kindness, 145
kink, 180, 196
knowledge, 13, 71, 153, 163, 173, 176, 188, 193, 196, 201, 203
Kolb, 153

lack, 21, 196
landscape, 126, 127, 131, 159, 183, 188, 193, 196
language, 21, 94, 103
lavender, 42, 56
layer, 60, 157
lead, 7, 9, 10, 12, 18, 54, 58, 59, 63, 70, 71, 76, 80, 84, 88, 101, 130, 131, 139, 143, 156, 158, 184, 186, 195
learning, 153, 156, 188, 192, 200
leash, 157
led, 179
legacy, 3
length, 70
lens, 179
level, 42, 47, 151
liberation, 5, 166
libido, 18
lie, 117, 164
life, 141
lifestyle, 15, 23, 25, 32, 40, 48, 54, 57, 62, 99, 112, 115, 126, 129, 143, 146, 148, 153, 155, 156, 158, 161, 162,

164, 174, 176, 183, 186–188, 190, 192, 193, 195, 196, 199, 201, 203, 208
light, 42, 59
lighting, 11, 41, 42, 48, 54
likelihood, 70
limelight, 180
limit, 100
lineage, 3, 179
list, 31, 177
listening, 31, 40
literature, 158, 173, 174, 176, 178, 180
location, 43–46, 48, 94, 127, 132, 136
look, 163, 164
loop, 4
love, 10, 18, 23, 69, 179
lung, 72

making, 11, 33, 42, 47, 49, 53, 75, 87, 151, 206
male, 12, 69, 70, 74, 75, 77
management, 135
manner, 1, 3, 5, 23, 131, 173, 199
mantra, 145
manual, 1
marriage, 179
massage, 55–57, 59
massager, 88
masturbation, 83
mating, 182
matter, 179
means, 31, 159, 180
meditation, 73
medium, 176
meet, 184
memorability, 28

memory, 42, 53
mentorship, 192
messiness, 59
method, 64, 78, 80, 180
mind, 70, 85, 95, 149, 156, 196
Mindfulness, 79
mindfulness, 70, 73, 92, 97, 98, 150, 161
mindset, 161
minute, 73
miscommunication, 160
misconception, 23, 24
misunderstanding, 23
mix, 19
model, 102
moment, 21, 40, 42, 60, 79, 97
monitoring, 101, 103, 112
mood, 42, 43, 50, 52
motherhood, 179
movement, 59
multitude, 146
muscle, 69
music, 42, 54, 151

narrative, 4
nature, 19, 24, 37, 42, 106, 109, 115, 129, 134, 180, 181, 184
navigation, 106
necessity, 128
need, 12, 102, 103, 129, 157, 184, 202
negotiation, 11, 19, 24, 37, 39, 40, 120, 134, 135
nerve, 75
networking, 186–188
niche, 184
noise, 42
non, 12, 21, 101, 110, 119, 129
normalization, 166, 180

nostalgia, 153
novice, 13
number, 31

observation, 103, 153
offering, 57, 67, 173, 176, 188
officer, 94
offspring, 179
on, 1–4, 10, 13, 16, 20, 23, 31, 37, 43, 48, 51, 58, 65, 67, 70, 72, 73, 75, 78, 79, 87–89, 98–100, 109, 110, 116, 118, 119, 135, 141, 144, 150–158, 163, 164, 173–177, 179–181, 186, 187, 196, 203
one, 3, 9, 10, 25, 28, 31, 37, 40, 73, 79, 83, 95, 99–101, 104, 109, 113, 118, 119, 127, 129, 139, 145, 150, 167, 186, 188, 199
opportunity, 37, 101, 117, 141, 143, 156, 163, 164, 195
orchestration, 64
orgasm, 64, 69, 70, 77–80, 85, 86
other, 16, 20, 31, 34, 39, 40, 47, 79, 99, 101, 102, 106, 118, 119, 145, 151, 157, 162
outlet, 150
overthinking, 79
ovulation, 203
oxytocin, 18, 69

page, 110, 135
painting, 150
park, 128
part, 4, 145, 155
participant, 13, 100, 129, 192
participation, 101, 109

partner, 4, 11, 28, 31, 32, 39, 40, 57, 62, 64, 78, 80, 88, 103, 118, 126, 155–157
party, 206, 208
passion, 19
past, 28, 151, 156, 163, 164
patch, 56
pathway, 57
patience, 160
pause, 28, 39, 100, 157, 159
penis, 58, 59, 78, 87
performance, 70, 73, 79, 80
perineum, 87
period, 70, 179
person, 4, 100, 104, 113, 184
persona, 157
perspective, 6, 17, 23, 24, 156
phase, 78, 80
phenomenon, 69, 71, 181
pheromone, 42
phrase, 100, 135
pinnacle, 3
place, 28, 48, 66, 119, 160
plan, 136, 155
planning, 129, 131, 132, 208
plateau, 78, 80
play, 16, 19, 42, 49, 53, 59, 67, 70, 77, 95, 96, 104, 109, 110, 112, 118, 128, 155, 162, 176, 183, 188, 199, 202, 208
playing, 92, 94
playlist, 42
pleasure, 7, 12, 13, 20, 37, 43, 46, 48, 49, 51, 54, 56–60, 62, 69–71, 74, 76, 77, 80, 82–88, 117, 118, 126, 132, 133, 146, 148, 156–158, 161, 164, 179, 204, 206

Index 219

plethora, 23, 184, 186
portrayal, 180
position, 59, 75
positivity, 5
possibility, 16, 70
post, 98, 101, 143, 149, 152
potential, 9, 10, 19, 20, 22, 32, 34, 38, 65, 67, 71, 75, 77, 79, 106, 116, 117, 119, 131, 134, 136, 137, 152, 162, 184–186, 196, 206, 208
power, 5, 18–20, 23, 36, 60, 96, 106, 113–116, 118–120, 123–126, 156, 163, 171, 173, 180, 190, 193, 196
practice, 9, 15, 17, 34, 57, 62, 75, 76, 78, 80, 98, 143, 145, 148, 151, 171, 181, 197
pregnancy, 20
preparation, 71, 92, 119, 158
presence, 134
pressure, 4, 56, 59, 70, 75, 78, 79, 84
principle, 21, 109
priority, 45
privacy, 43, 46, 48, 131, 134–136
process, 9, 10, 27, 29, 37, 58, 60, 66, 77, 80, 98, 104, 109, 119, 129, 138, 141, 145, 149, 153–156, 158, 188
processing, 12, 150
procreation, 23
professional, 146–148, 150, 199
progress, 73
property, 179
prostate, 12, 70, 75–77, 87, 88, 157
protector, 179
prowess, 5
psychology, 18–20, 48, 181

public, 17, 18, 22, 24, 31, 109–112, 127–139, 156
purpose, 162, 179
pursuit, 7, 183

quality, 182, 205
quantity, 182
question, 21, 31

range, 2, 12, 16, 23, 87, 129, 132, 143, 157, 174, 194
rate, 69, 80
readiness, 158, 159
reality, 23
realm, 10, 27, 30, 32, 34, 46, 57, 86, 92, 95, 99, 101, 106, 109, 113, 127, 148, 156, 158, 171, 188, 193, 201, 204
reassurance, 188
receiver, 56
reclamation, 180
recovery, 6, 10, 73
rectum, 75
red, 103
Reddit, 192
reflection, 39, 101, 125, 153–156, 158, 159, 163
regimen, 74
relation, 180
relationship, 23, 47, 113, 150, 162, 180, 199
relaxation, 11, 42, 56, 57, 79
release, 18, 65, 69, 80, 82
removal, 47
repository, 192
reproduction, 3, 4, 179–181
research, 183
resilience, 150
resistance, 180

resolution, 134
resource, 1, 3, 13, 178
respect, 22–24, 29, 34, 103, 104, 106, 109, 120, 127, 129, 132, 136
response, 18, 70, 71, 77, 129
responsibility, 119
restraint, 80
return, 141
revocability, 21
right, 12, 41, 43, 46, 48, 50, 86, 87, 136, 196, 199, 200, 204, 206
rise, 166, 180
risk, 94, 100, 130
role, 4, 11, 16, 42, 43, 49, 53, 67, 69, 70, 75, 85, 92, 94–96, 104, 110, 118, 128, 156, 157, 162, 188, 196, 199, 202, 206, 208
roleplay, 9, 39, 60, 65–67, 85, 152, 157, 163
roleplaying, 60
romance, 42
room, 42
routine, 57, 73, 148, 149
running, 72

s, 3, 6, 11, 18, 25, 31, 34, 48, 70, 77, 79, 83, 99, 102–104, 106, 139, 151, 153, 180, 188, 199, 203, 205, 208
safety, 4, 12, 13, 18, 20, 23–25, 27, 30, 32–34, 45, 46, 48, 50, 88–92, 117, 126, 129, 131, 132, 135, 139, 151, 156–161, 201, 205, 206
saliva, 59

satisfaction, 5, 8, 9, 18, 48, 65, 74, 92, 112, 150, 156–161, 164
scenario, 19, 88, 94, 128, 157
scene, 4, 9, 11, 15, 16, 18, 20, 28, 31, 34, 37–42, 51, 54, 60, 91, 94, 100–103, 105, 110, 118, 119, 128–130, 132, 135, 141–143, 145, 149, 150, 152, 155, 157, 159, 160
scent, 41, 42, 48
science, 6, 69, 71
score, 73
scrutiny, 24
search, 185
section, 5, 8, 15, 20, 23, 30, 32, 34, 37, 41, 43, 46, 48, 51, 55, 58, 60, 63, 65, 71, 74, 77, 83, 86, 89, 92, 95, 99, 101, 106, 115, 118, 129, 132, 134, 137, 143, 150, 153, 156, 158, 162, 171, 176, 179, 181, 184, 186, 188, 191, 196, 199, 204, 206
secure, 10, 19, 24, 137, 151, 158
security, 18, 45, 157
selection, 46, 181
self, 5, 17, 83–86, 92, 98, 125, 126, 145, 148, 150, 153, 156, 159, 188
sensation, 56
sense, 5, 8, 9, 11, 16, 20, 27, 49, 50, 52, 53, 57, 63, 87, 95, 97, 98, 131, 133, 150, 152, 155, 183, 188, 193, 196
sensitivity, 59, 80
sensuality, 42
series, 69

service, 205
session, 11, 39, 88, 89, 142, 196
set, 11, 37, 42, 94, 104, 157
setting, 11, 28, 31, 43, 48, 60, 129, 132, 160, 162, 164, 188, 192
sex, 4, 199–203
sexuality, 1, 3–5, 22, 24, 69, 71, 137, 150, 162, 175, 176, 179–181, 183, 199
shaft, 59
shame, 86, 142, 150, 199
shape, 181
share, 28, 31, 40, 137, 145, 150, 163, 166, 184, 186, 188, 189
sharing, 30, 149, 188–190, 192
shift, 21, 37, 40, 156, 179
sight, 47, 51, 54
sign, 148
signal, 28, 135, 157, 159
significance, 5, 15, 27, 41, 99, 141, 176, 179–181, 196, 199
situation, 40, 99, 129, 155
skill, 79
skin, 57
smell, 51, 53, 54
society, 4, 23, 25, 167, 179, 180
solo, 17, 18, 77, 86–98
sound, 41, 48, 51, 54
space, 11, 12, 23, 24, 41–43, 48, 50–52, 54, 94, 104, 120, 129, 131, 132, 150, 151, 156, 176, 189, 191, 196
specialist, 203
spectrum, 7, 148
speed, 59, 88
sperm, 75
spirit, 95
spot, 70, 74

sprint, 73
squeeze, 78, 80
stage, 11, 30, 48, 94, 153
stamina, 71–74
start, 78, 80
step, 29, 30, 32, 37, 65, 127, 146, 148, 164, 199
stereotype, 23
stigma, 24
stimulation, 12, 17, 52, 54, 58–60, 70, 74–78, 80, 83–88, 157
stone, 37
stop, 28, 78, 80, 100, 159
story, 150
storytelling, 189
strength, 73
stress, 70
stroker, 88
structure, 11
subject, 69, 162
submission, 3, 19, 47, 115
submissive, 4, 19, 23, 94, 103, 118, 123, 156, 157
success, 117, 181, 206, 208
succession, 70
suit, 94
summary, 3, 13, 22, 71
sun, 43
support, 37, 80, 145–148, 150, 160, 167, 183, 188, 196, 199, 202
surface, 56, 66
surrounding, 3, 24, 127, 171, 180, 181
survival, 3
swimming, 72
system, 69, 75

t, 157

taboo, 3, 23, 30
tailor, 84
talk, 60–62
tap, 3, 18
tapestry, 5, 15, 48, 95, 164, 181, 183
taste, 51, 54
teasing, 65
technique, 31, 78, 80, 82, 149
television, 180
temperature, 41, 42, 57
tension, 69
territory, 27
test, 56
testing, 24, 203
theory, 18, 30, 48, 150, 153, 171, 181
therapist, 145, 198
therapy, 150, 196, 199
thought, 17, 79
thoughtfulness, 48
thrill, 17, 19, 24, 94, 112, 131, 132, 136, 156
time, 20, 21, 34, 98, 101, 119, 152, 154, 158, 165
tongue, 59
tool, 53, 57, 100, 135, 156, 157, 176
touch, 47, 50–52, 54, 59, 65, 75, 100
toy, 87, 88, 205
track, 154
tracking, 203
training, 73, 74
transformation, 153
traveler, 94
trigger, 18, 47
triggers, 66
trust, 4, 8, 10, 11, 15, 18, 20, 23, 29, 30, 33, 34, 37, 47, 113, 115, 116, 120, 126, 145, 149–152, 155, 158, 160, 189, 190
truth, 95
turbulence, 145
type, 15, 16, 70

understanding, 1, 3, 7, 9, 10, 12, 20, 22–24, 34, 37, 47, 48, 57, 60, 62, 67, 71, 77, 82, 87, 101, 106, 109, 110, 117, 124, 126–129, 131, 137, 139, 145, 150, 152, 153, 156, 158, 160, 164–166, 171, 173, 174, 176, 178, 181, 183, 190, 192, 193, 196, 208
uniform, 94
unity, 9, 57
up, 152
urge, 18, 19
use, 11, 24, 42, 46, 47, 49, 59, 94, 100, 103, 157
user, 88

validation, 188
variety, 15, 158
vehicle, 3
venue, 48
view, 24, 100
vigilance, 104
violation, 129
visibility, 109, 136
visualization, 70
voice, 38
vulnerability, 3, 4, 20, 22, 24, 101, 113, 123, 134, 143, 146, 148, 152
vulva, 58

walking, 73

wall, 75
walnut, 75
warm, 42, 57, 59, 149, 152
warmth, 42, 43
way, 40, 55, 83, 98, 145, 164, 166, 196
weakness, 148
wealth, 163, 173
webinar, 194
website, 192
week, 72
well, 12, 13, 16, 32, 34, 48, 99, 101, 127, 142, 145, 146, 148, 153, 155, 157, 158, 161, 174, 190, 196, 201, 204

wellness, 148–150, 166, 174, 175, 201, 203
whole, 192
willingness, 10, 21, 82, 156, 196
wine, 31
wisdom, 190
withdrawal, 21
word, 28, 39, 40, 100, 103, 135, 157, 159
work, 175
workout, 73
workshop, 194
world, 3, 71, 112, 178, 196, 206
worry, 59
writing, 150